WHEN TWO LOVES COLLIDE

With warmest regards,

[signature]

[signature]

When Two Loves Collide

THE INSPIRING STORY OF
DR. JOHN AND DOT MOONEY

William G. Borchert

Tasora

A portion of the proceeds from this book will be donated to
The National Council on Alcoholism and Drug Dependence.

———————————

Tasora Books
5120 Cedar Lake Road
Minneapolis, MN 55416
(952) 345-4488

Distributed by Itascia Books

Printed in Canada on acid-free paper.

ISBN: 978-1-934690-61-1

Cover design by Rachel Mooney Spence

To order additional copies of this book, please go to:
www.itascabooks.com

To my dear wife, Bernadette . . .
for her long and loving commitment.

CONTENTS

AUTHOR'S NOTE

THERE ARE TIMES IN AN AUTHOR'S LIFE WHEN HE FEELS TRULY privileged to have the opportunity to write a particular story— usually when that story involves exceptional people who have done exceptional things—and seek no credit in return.

The writing of this book, *When Two Loves Collide,* is one of those special times for this author.

This story embraces the deeply passionate and committed relationship between a heroic, battle-scarred army surgeon and a warm and beautiful Georgia country girl who, together, faced their demons and won. As a result of their painful and often near-disastrous struggle, they were able to help countless others also find the road to redemption and recovery.

In the end, it was the force of their strong and unwavering commitment to each other—even in the worst of times—that enabled them to discover a kind of life they never dreamed possible and to share that life with so many others.

Dr. John Mooney and his wife, Dot, had the kind of commitment we do not find very often today. The word "commitment" was once almost synonymous with a sacred oath. It was the grip of a handshake that closed a deal, the anvil of confidence that brought things to fruition. Most of all, it was the mortar that so-lidified relationships, the one thing that made them strong, whole, and lasting. It was the virtue that engendered hope and faith in the idea that tomorrow would be a better day.

A true commitment is still what transforms a promise into re-ality. It is what boldly clarifies your intentions and makes your ac-tions speak louder than your words. It is making the time when there is none . . . coming through time after time . . . year after year after year.

Commitment is the stuff character is made of, for it has the power to change the very face of things. It is the daily triumph of integrity over skepticism. For Dot and John Mooney, it meant . . . when I say I love you, I mean I'm committed to working to love you even when it's hard to do.

But that was then and this is now. It's sad to see that something has happened to the meaning of that word since then. It has lost some of its luster, some of its pride, some of its reverence. It has become limp and, at times, deceptive. For many in this day and age, true commitment is no longer one of the most essential in-gredients in our character even though it is an ingredient that af-fects every aspect of our lives.

It is my hope that in telling the story of Dr. John Mooney and his loving wife, Dot, many will come to realize that unless we stand by our commitments, those we make both to ourselves and to others, we could well begin to doubt the worth of our lives, forget how to love unconditionally, lose hope and faith in the fu-ture, give up too soon, and thus never realize the fulfillment of our dreams.

As Dot Mooney used to say to anyone who would listen, "Please don't give up before the dream happens. For it surely will."

FOREWORD

Claudia Black

HOW DO YOU GO FROM BEING A SKILLED, ADMIRED SURGEON and a decorated World War II veteran to being Dr. 58520, prisoner in the U.S. Federal Narcotics Prison in Lexington, Kentucky? How do you go from being a fun-loving, bright, passionate nurse to a desperate woman with suicidal thoughts and the "Georgia power cocktail"—electric shock therapy? For John Mooney and his wife, Dot, the how and why were complex, and yet one word summed it up—addiction.

How do you get back from the Georgia power cocktail and federal prison to not only finding an answer for yourself but one that continues to save thousands of other lives? That is their remarkable story.

Dot and John journeyed into their addictions separately, but their journeys reflect the universality of the progression of the disease for two people who came from very different backgrounds. From the start, they loved each other passionately. But soon they came to love their addictions almost as passionately . . . and when those two loves collided, the result was chaos.

Dot was a farm girl who loved the country life. A fun-loving and popular teenager, she was also rebelling against a strict mom. She loved to roll up the rugs and dance with friends for hours to records played on her Victrola. This was the backdrop to Dot's first magical experience with alcohol. Although she would throw up and have a hangover, what she remembered most was the "thrill of flying through the great, blue Carolina skies and the contentment that comes from being so happily at peace with the world and everyone in it."

The son of a highly respected physician, John grew up with the privileges of greater economic security and the expectation that he too would be successful. His family members abstained from alcohol in the era when one who did so was called a teetotaler, often having been preached to about "the evils of drinking." While John grew up believing that drinking alcohol was something you didn't do, he was titillated by the fun times he saw others having once he was in college. He was hooked by his initial experience: "As soon as alcohol reached my brain, it put me off into another world. I would live in that world for the next thirty years. I used to think it took a long time to become an alcoholic. That night it took me about one minute and forty-five seconds."

While this story begins with Dot and John coming of age as the world was entering into World War II, it is a story that has been replicated throughout the generations. A young man and woman fall madly in love and want to live the American dream of creating a family and making a contribution in their community. As a part of life, they do what most adult Americans do, they drink. They begin their drinking for much the same reasons others choose to drink. It looks like fun; it's the adult thing to do. And they, like approximately 10 percent of others who choose to drink, find alcohol does something for them it doesn't necessarily do for others. It fills a hole they may never have known they had.

When Two Loves Collide describes the irrational yet recognizable behavior of people who need to drink to feel normal. It shows the common defenses of justifying, rationalizing, and denying, defenses that fuel and sustain addiction. You will see how Dot and John became perfectionists in the art of self-deception.

From the havoc of these two devastated lives, and buoyed by a loving commitment to each other that was the centerpiece of their relationship, the Mooneys would find their way out of their combined horrors. Unfortunately, before that could happen, their torment would touch their children.

While some people want to believe children are not affected, the truth is, they are. Certainly the degree to which children are affected varies. You will read how the three sons born into their parents' active illness each had different experiences. There were good as well as painful times. As much as these two parents wanted and genuinely loved their children, their problems strongly interfered with healthy parenting.

The young boys would listen to their parents argue night after night and then the next morning act as if everything was okay. Their feelings were discounted when they were told they had nothing to be afraid of—in reality they had much to be afraid of. They listened to their parents lie, make excuses, and be dishonest in other ways. Other kids were not invited to play at their home. Dad disappeared for long periods of time with vague excuses being offered for his whereabouts. All three boys describe the inconsistencies of their parents' behavior. For the most part they knew they were loved, but were confused by the irrational and often painful behavior they observed.

Today it is recognized that people seek help for their addiction when they reach their bottom. But what we also now recognize is that "bottom" has a different meaning for each person. For some, it is the first embarrassing scene that takes place at a social event; for another it is with the first, or the fifth, DUI, or when a friend confronts them about their using. But sadly, for the majority, their path is similar to that of the Mooneys. When they can't find a way to go any further in life other than the proverbial "jails, institutions, or death," the answer comes to them. They begin to experience moments of honesty with themselves that ultimately lead them to the realization that they are powerless and that their lives are completely unmanageable . . . and find their answers in a Twelve-Step program like Alcoholics Anonymous.

At that point in their lives, Dot and John demonstrated what is necessary to find recovery. They were willing to go to any lengths. They found recovery in AA's Twelve-Step program, and their entire family began to get well.

Experiencing great gratitude, they felt a passion about extending their recovery to others. It soon became their life focus. At first, they opened their home to those who were seriously sick and in need of detoxification. Within a few years, while believing the Twelve-Step programs worked, they also came to recognize that some people were so sick, they needed more, and they opened one of the earliest treatment hospitals in our country dedicated to the physical, mental, and spiritual components of recovery.

Believing that "if you are willing, there is a way," they founded Willingway, which opened its doors in 1971. Steeped in the principles of Twelve-Step recovery, it continues today to be nationally known for utilizing abstinence, not medication-based treatment. John and Dot Mooney had learned the hard way that there were no safe, nonaddictive medications for most alcoholics and drug addicts.

While Dot and John passionately began to tend to the sick addicts sharing their home, their family continued to grow. In addition to their three boys, they welcomed a baby girl—born into a family that was now in recovery.

It has been said that "once you see addiction in a family, look again." Fortunately all four of the Mooney children found recovery for themselves. Not only that, they have followed in the footsteps of their sober parents. Each of the Mooney children—from Al to Jimmy, Bobby, and Carol Lind—has continued in that path. They have dedicated their lives—both personally and professionally—to the recovery of alcoholics and drug addicts, family members as well as active participants at Willingway.

The story recounted in *When Two Loves Collide* spans decades, giving the reader a historical perspective of the evolution of treatment. In the past, many who suffered with addiction were treated with electric shock therapy, or given paraldehyde, a drug so toxic it had to be banned from use. For years people with addiction were placed in asylums if they were poor and sanitariums if they were wealthy. To this day, many are incarcerated in prison. The stigma they felt is still experienced today, sixty years later. Individuals, couples, and families go to great lengths not to name addiction for what it is—a progressive disease. Rather, they justify, rationalize, and blatantly deny—and the disease progresses.

Addiction is said to be an equal opportunity destroyer. It can and does have an impact on men and women, the young and the old, the less and the better educated, the impoverished and the wealthy. It crosses into all races and religious affiliations. And it is experienced in at least one out of every four families. The good news is, as devastating as it is, recovery is possible.

Dot and John Mooney have now passed away, but what they would want the reader to know is that there is hope for recovery from this illness for both the alcoholic and the addict—and for his or her family, since this is truly a family disease. Recovery is the road back to integrity and dignity, to self-love and the love of others.

When Two Loves Collide is an incredibly inspirational story and a touching and beautiful legacy.

CLAUDIA BLACK is a nationally known addiction specialist and acclaimed author of many books, including *It Will Never Happen to Me: Growing Up with Addiction as Youngsters, Adolescents, Adults*; *Changing Course: Healing from Loss, Abandonment, and Fear*; and *My Dad Loves Me, My Dad Has a Disease; A Child's View: Living with Addiction*.

ACKNOWLEDGMENTS

THE AUTHOR WOULD LIKE TO EXPRESS HIS GRATITUDE AND deep appreciation to all those who gave so generously of their time, their thoughts, and their guidance to help make this book possible.

The primary source of the factual material contained in this book came from the frequent talks that the late Dr. John Mooney and his wife, Dot Mooney, gave at meetings and conventions of Alcoholics Anonymous, addiction treatment seminars, and medical conferences, many of which were taped and transcribed.

The second important source of factual information was from the historical accounts and in-depth interviews the author had with the late couple's four children: Dr. Al Mooney, Jimmy Mooney, Dr. Robert Mooney, and Carol Lind Mooney, all of whom approved the final manuscript.

Their accounts and recollections were further expanded upon and substantiated by in-depth interviews with more than thirty other surviving family members and close personal friends of the late physician and his wife. These included Dr. John Mooney's office nurse of many years, Dallas Cason, and his friend and accountant,

Earl Dabbs, who helped make possible the doctor's dream of saving thousands of alcoholics and drug addicts.

Other important sources included the personal journal of the late Professor Jack Averitt of Georgia Southern University, a dear friend who helped John and Dot Mooney find a solution to their disease; newspaper, magazine, and medical journal articles written about Dr. Mooney's life and discoveries; reports from the U.S. Public Health Narcotics Prison in Lexington, Kentucky, where the late physician was sentenced for a drug felony charge; newspaper columns and other stories written by Dr. Mooney; and lengthy research into the historical times, places, and significant events that touched the lives of this important couple.

The author would also like to extend his special thanks to Mrs. Robbin Mooney for her assistance in arranging important meetings and interviews to gather data and necessary information and for her significant effort in researching certain events, times, and places important to this story.

The cover of the book was designed by Rachel Mooney Spence, granddaughter of Dr. John and Dot Mooney and the head of Designatorium.com.

Willingway, the institution founded by Dr. John and Dot Mooney in Statesboro, Georgia, continues to live on in their memory, saving the lives of thousands of alcoholics and drug addicts, and healing families affected by this terrible disease.

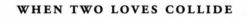

WHEN TWO LOVES COLLIDE

CHAPTER ONE

"Doctor 58520"

IT WAS A NIGHT HE WOULD NEVER FORGET . . . FROM THE MO-ment he heard the steel cell door slam shut behind him to the twitch in his nostrils from the dank smell that filled the small, clammy cubicle.

He was in prison—the U.S. Federal Narcotics Prison in Lexington, Kentucky. It was July 13, 1959, and Dr. Alfonso John Mooney Jr., a war hero, a renowned surgeon, and a proud husband and father, was now a common criminal convicted of trafficking in narcotics and using illegal and prescription drugs.

His hands shook as he tossed his bedroll onto the bunk hanging from chains drilled into the peeling cement wall. He stood there trying to stop his befogged brain from racing through ungraspable thoughts, trying to grab on to just one that might explain why a man like himself—an intelligent, skilled, and once highly respected doctor—had reached such a hellish, shameful, unbelievable bottom in his life.

As he stared down at his gray prison garb with black numbers stamped on the front and back of the wrinkled jacket, he suddenly realized he was no longer Dr. John Mooney Jr., the well-known surgeon from Statesboro, Georgia. He was now "Dr. 58520," a convicted drug felon.

After standing there for a long moment, he walked slowly to the barred window at the other end of his cell and looked out. A tall lamppost in the prison yard cast a pale glow on his face. His once-handsome features were now marred by red blotches and a stubble of beard that belied his age of forty-nine. He looked at least twenty years older. His once sparkling blue eyes were now red and sad, and his strapping shoulders sagged beneath the weight of his despair.

I'm Doctor John Mooney, he kept murmuring to himself. I'm not a bad person. I'm not a criminal. Why am I in prison? The only response he heard was from the crickets and other insects buzzing around free outside his cell window.

John was not only in prison, he was in one of the most notorious prisons in the entire federal penitentiary system. Lexington, however, wasn't notorious because it housed the worst killers, robbers, and rapists in the country. It didn't. It was notorious because of its uniqueness and controversial reputation.

The United States Federal Narcotics Prison was one of those grand American experiments—a multi-million-dollar attempt to solve the nation's drug addiction problem and reduce the crime rate resulting from illegal drugs. Eager politicians thought it could be done through judicial punishment for criminal offenses, social rehabilitation, and recovery from drug addiction through medical and psychiatric treatment.

In 1929, when the U.S. Congress authorized the U.S. Public Health Service to join with the federal penitentiary system to establish the narcotics prison, the only such facility in the world at the time, its stated purpose was "for the confinement and treatment of persons addicted to the use of habit-forming narcotic drugs."

The sprawling 1,050-acre site located in the rolling hills of Kentucky was built and run like a minimum-security prison with both cells and dorms and steel gates and barred windows. There were also well-equipped prison guards to handle the outbreaks of sudden rage from drug withdrawals or the cutoff of privileges, as well as the hallucinations and convulsions usually associated with the newer arrivals. While the high walls guarded the ominous-looking buildings on the inside, there was a prison farm and dairy on the outside where many of the inmates worked. It was thought to be therapeutic for them to hoe the ground, milk the cows, and shovel the manure.

While John Mooney didn't find himself in the company of hard-core killers and rapists, he did find himself in the company of some of the more notorious celebrities from the world of arts and entertainment.

The famous actor Peter Lorre was incarcerated at the Lexington federal prison for his addiction to morphine. Best known for playing strange and sinister roles, the Hungarian-born character actor starred in such movies as *Casablanca, The Maltese Falcon,* and *Arsenic and Old Lace.* He never recovered from his drug addiction. Neither did legendary jazz musicians Sonny Rollins and Chet Baker, two more of the many celebrated, drug-addicted artists who came through the Lexington, Kentucky, prison/hospital facility.

Some guards and nurses who once worked at the controversial institution claimed the doctors used untested treatments such as risky, unproven medications to block the action of opiates. Other doctors were said to have bribed prisoners with heroin and cocaine so they would be "guinea pigs" for bizarre and highly questionable experiments.

A full-scale congressional investigation that led to the eventual closing of the Lexington narcotics prison discovered that many of these "bribed" inmates were stripped of their clothing while high on drugs and had their pubic hair burned off. Other male prisoners had their genitals placed in ice water for long periods of time in an attempt to reduce their craving for narcotics.

But as "Dr. 58520" continued to stare through the steel bars of his jail cell window that night, he was completely unaware that any of these bizarre forms of drug addiction treatments could be awaiting him. He only knew that he had never felt so totally alone before . . . so lost and bewildered . . . so filled with fear and guilt. Not only had he devastated his own family, but just the week before his mother had died . . . and he was drunk. He hadn't seen her in some time. He wasn't even with her or even near her when she passed away. He was under arrest, waiting for his future to be decided by the courts.

Now he felt like he himself was dying . . . dying inside. Or maybe it was more like he was hoping to die . . . that he had nothing left to live for . . . that everything near and dear to him in life was gone. That he had lost it all or given it away for another drink or another drug.

People who have had near-death experiences say that their whole life flashes before them. It happened to John Mooney that night.

He turned away from the window, walked slowly to his bunk, and sat down on the hard, thin mattress. As he stared at the floor, he began to think about his beautiful wife, Dot, the only person who ever made him feel really loved. All his life he wanted to feel loved, but it never happened . . . not until Dorothy Riggs came into his life. She filled him with passion, with desire, with wanting to be near her and always thinking of her when they were apart. That is . . . until their demons tried to tear them from each other's arms.

But then their children drew them back together, three wonderful sons who came along in quick succession. That made things all right for a while. Still, the demons of addiction never let up. They invade every aspect of your life . . . leave no stone unturned. They stole his family, his income, his career, his life savings, even his God, leaving him physically, mentally, and spiritually bankrupt. Prayer was like ashes on his tongue. They take and they take until there is no more to be taken. And then they bring you here . . . to a hell on earth. He shook his head.

He began to think of his mother, how she had always tried to protect him, perhaps too much. As John's childhood now began to flash in front of him . . . his friends . . . his growing-up years—he was suddenly startled by a shrill whistle that echoed through the cell block. The whistle was followed by a forceful voice shouting, "Lights out! All lights out!"

The single lightbulb in the ceiling above him flickered, then went out. Only the tall lamppost in the prison yard filled John's cell with a dim glow. He lay down on his bunk, resting his head on his bedroll, listening to the strange, hushed sounds that surrounded him. Then the sounds gradually became recognizable . . . like voices in his head . . . voices that had been haunting him since this whole nightmare of his arrest, conviction, and incarceration began.

He could hear the voice of Bulloch County, Georgia Judge Robert Mikell:

> "Heretofore a lunacy warrant has been issued from this court for the arrest of John Mooney, Jr., and he having been arrested is confined for safe keeping in St. Joseph's Hospital in Savannah, Georgia until further order of this court.
>
> "And, said John Mooney, Jr.'s mother, having this day, July 7, 1959, passed away and it is the desire of the family that he be allowed to leave the confines of said hospital to attend his mother's funeral, it is ordered that the said John Mooney, Jr., be temporarily released into the custody of any sheriff or deputy of this state for the purpose of attending his mother's funeral in Statesboro, Georgia, and immediately after said funeral the said John Mooney, Jr., is to be returned to said hospital and placed in confinement and safely held until further order of this court."

As Judge Mikell's voice faded away, John heard the voice of Georgia Superior Court Judge J. L. Renfroe:

"Whereupon, on this day of July 10, 1959, it is the judgment of the court that you, John Mooney, Jr., be taken from the Court House to the common jail of Bulloch County and be kept in safe custody till remanded by a guard from the Penitentiary, and be taken hence by said guard to the Federal Penitentiary in Reidsville, Georgia or such other place as the Governor shall direct and be there confined to hard labor for the space of not less than two years nor more than two years, and then be discharged.

"This sentence is hereby probated, however, upon you being confined at the U.S. Narcotics Prison in Lexington, Kentucky where you will remain and be treated for drug addiction until you are pronounced cured."

John had known James Renfroe long before he became a judge. He knew him when they were growing up in Statesboro and when he became a lawyer. The judge was good friends with his mother and father. He thought he was also his friend. But now in his befogged brain, John hated Superior Court Judge J. L. Renfroe for sending him to prison. At the same time, however, he knew deep in his heart that with the felony drug charges against him, the judge's hands were tied. That sending him to Lexington for treatment instead of to the maximum-security federal penitentiary in Reidsville was the best thing he could do for a doctor he once respected.

For some reason, all of these thoughts brought to mind what was going to happen the next day, something he had better prepare for. Like all newly confined drug addicts, he was going before the prison/hospital's psychiatric board for a full psychiatric evaluation.

Perhaps if they find I'm not a complete raving lunatic, he thought—even if my arrest warrant says otherwise—they might transition me into the dormitory population. There I would at least have more freedom to move about, to talk with fellow inmates, and not feel like Al Capone in solitary confinement.

I'll put on the best show I can, he said to himself. Then, a moment later, he realized he had been doing that for most of his life. Putting on a show wasn't working anymore. In fact, as much as he didn't want to admit it, it was his best acting and his best thinking that finally landed him in here. Maybe this time, he ought to let things just happen the way they're supposed to happen.

By now he was exhausted, mentally and physically. As he closed his eyes and hoped for some sleep, he heard one more voice in his head. It was a voice he needed to hear—at least tonight. It was Dot's voice: *I love you, John. I love you with all my heart. Nothing will ever stop me from loving you. Nothing.*

CHAPTER TWO

A Challenge from the Start

JOHN MOONEY JR. WAS BORN INTO A FAMILY OF QUITE COM-
fortable means. His father was a respected country doctor, his
mother a strong, churchgoing woman, and he was right in the
middle of two attractive sisters, who could be sweet to him one
minute and mean to him the next. But he came to love them
both.

It was March 14, 1910, when John first opened his eyes in the
warmth of his mother's arms in Bulloch County Hospital in
the small but thriving city of Statesboro, Georgia. America was
booming then, as was "King Cotton" in Georgia. So he found
himself entering a world that could offer him almost anything
he could possibly want and certainly everything he would need.
Yet, even before he could crawl, toddle, or mumble his first words,
John Mooney wanted more. He wanted more of everything.

This character trait would become for a while the cornerstone
of his personality, the fuel for his great success, and, sadly, the
eventual pathway to failure and disgrace. It would be diagnosed

later in life as "a strong tendency towards excesses resulting from a need to over-compensate."

Perhaps, at least in the beginning, it was an understandable trait since "over-compensation" was one of the ways—as a young boy at least—that John dealt with his rather significant and burdensome inferiority complex.

John Mooney was born with a nevus on his face, a congenital, pigmented lesion that marred his good looks and, as he grew older, drew unwanted attention from playmates and children at school. His father, Dr. Alfonso John Mooney Sr., a skilled doctor who was also the city physician for Statesboro, decided it would be best not to have the facial lesion removed until his son was a bit older and his features had filled out somewhat. His mother, Sallie Ethel Wimberly Mooney, agreed with her husband once she understood how much better the outcome could possibly be if the procedure were done at a somewhat older age.

But young John didn't agree. He couldn't seem to get his parents to understand how painful it was just to go out and play or to go to school. Wherever he went, there were always those funny looks, those hidden snickers. It made him feel like less of a person, almost like some kind of a circus freak. The truth is, the nevus wasn't nearly as bad as what the young boy saw when looking into a mirror. But it sorely affected his self-esteem and created a deep inferiority complex, something his parents were late to recognize.

Despite their son's constant pleas, sullen moods, and angry accusations that they did not love him, Dr. and Mrs. Mooney waited until John was ten before having a specialist perform what turned out to be a very successful surgical outcome. It left the boy with an almost unnoticeable scar and a brand-new zest for life.

The same year he turned ten, a major influenza epidemic broke out in Statesboro, taking the lives of a number its citizens. There were no flu shots or efficacious medicines to treat influenza at the time so, as city physician, Dr. Mooney ordered that all public gathering places be shut down. These included churches, schools, social clubs, lodge meetings, and movie theaters. The ban lasted for well over a month while Dr. Mooney reviewed all the flu and pneumonia cases at the overcrowded hospital and at a hotel on Main Street where the overflow cases were sent. His son and daughters enjoyed the month off from school. John in particular enjoyed it since he had now been accepted by a growing list of friends.

While few noticed the small scar on John's face, the scars on the inside from all the perceived and imagined ridicule were still there. And it wasn't only those hurtful barbs. Before the removal of his facial blemish, John's parents were very concerned about any physical injury to the lesion and therefore were very protective of him—at times, overprotective. He was not allowed to play any rough-and-tumble games or sports such as football. So he began to read a lot and soon discovered he was nearsighted and needed glasses. This only added to his feelings of being different and less than.

In addition to reading, John fell in love with music, all kinds of music. It made him feel comfortable, at ease, and took him out of himself. Then he learned to play the violin and soon was playing it well and at school concerts. This bolstered his ego a bit, together with the excellent grades he was receiving in all his subjects.

In addition to being exceptionally studious, the young boy also developed deep religious convictions and a strong faith in God, much of this having to do with his parents, who were both dedicated Christian people. Sallie Mooney was a superintendent of the Junior Sunday School in the Methodist church while his father was on the Board of Deacons in the Baptist church.

Despite the fact that it was a family of divided Christianity and some strong philosophical differences, there was usually harmony at the dinner table and a commitment to family prayer every evening. Together with his sisters, John would kneel down each night while his father read from the Bible and their mother led them in prayer.

It was also due in part to their Christian belief system that there was never any alcohol in the house. His parents didn't drink, and John never saw anyone in his extended family or any visitors to their home ever touch a drop of liquor. Perhaps that's why the young boy got the idea that decent people didn't drink. All through high school he didn't believe anyone should drink and looked down upon people who did.

Young John began to hit his stride after the successful surgery on his face. As he grew into his teen years, the city of Statesboro continued to grow up with him. What fueled its expansion was cotton. For example, the year John Mooney was born, Statesboro led the world in the sales of long-staple Sea Island cotton. For each bale of cotton sold in Savannah, ten bales were sold in Statesboro.

As it turned out, Doctor Mooney was not only a fine physician, he was also a shrewd businessman. He became a heavy investor in cotton and later in another major cash crop, tobacco, which flourished in the rich soil in and around Statesboro. With the profits he made, Dr. Mooney joined with several of his wealthy friends to open a bank in the city, the Bank of Statesboro, which helped farmers finance and harvest their crops.

As the wealth of the city grew and more people moved in, there was a greater need for better infrastructure, including roads, housing, schools, and other services. Young John was approaching high school age when the city council proposed a big bond referendum to build a new and much larger high school. It was passed and the school was completed just in time for the teenager to start his freshman year. The following year, the Women's Club of Statesboro built the city's first public library, and he spent hours there devouring its books.

A major event occurred in Statesboro during John's junior year in high school. The city council acknowledged its responsibility to provide educational opportunities to all the children in the community and voted unanimously to build a school for the black children. It was initially a one-story brick veneer building that cost the taxpayers $10,000. It was later expanded and a new black high school was built as well.

By the time John Mooney Jr. became a senior at Statesboro High, the now tall and very good-looking young man had become one of the more popular members of his class, a real ladies man and a "go-to guy" for those who were having difficulty with their studies. He was considered "a brain," which back then was a respected term when compared to what a "nerd" is today. He graduated early, at age sixteen, and with honors. He now had a great deal more self-confidence, which was slowly chipping away at his lingering inferiority complex.

Since Dr. Mooney was a fourth-generation physician, it was only natural that he would want his son to follow in his footsteps. He was very pleased when John began showing an inclination in that direction. In fact, John's favorite subject in high school was biology. Also, he was now constantly asking his father more than just curious questions about his practice—the kinds of difficult cases he was getting at his office and at the hospital and how he was treating them.

It was about a year before John's high school graduation that the doctor and his son began talking seriously about medical school and what were the best ones in Georgia. A short time later they started visiting a few in Savannah, Macon, and Atlanta. The city physician of Statesboro was once again very pleased when his son decided to attend Emory University School of Medicine in Atlanta. Emory was known as Atlanta Medical College during Dr. Mooney's time there as a student, and he was amazed at how much the school had progressed since he received his medical degree. Today it is one of the top twenty medical schools in the country.

Over the course of the Mooney family's four generations in

medicine, the heroic art of healing had changed dramatically. And Emory University, which dates back to February 14, 1854, helped bring medicine into the modern age by establishing a formal training curriculum for those choosing to become doctors.

It was on that date in 1854 when a group of Atlanta physicians, supported by the Georgia legislature, joined together to launch one of the very first schools that would supply adequate facilities for clinical instruction. Prior to this, there were much quackery and homemade remedies and so-called medical clinics that taught the fads and the fancies of the day. This usually meant the three basic principles most doctors accepted at the turn of the century: bloodletting, blistering, and purgation. And many so-called physicians practiced without any formal training other than being an apprentice to another poorly trained physician.

But Emory, like others to follow, changed all of that. The university's goal was to join the best cutting-edge technology and world-class research to patient-centered and socially conscious clinical training. From those early beginnings as a small, struggling program, Emory has emerged today as one of the more innovative medical centers in the land.

One of the more important accomplishments in the early years of Emory's growth was the establishment of a close working relationship and the eventual merging of its medical programs with Grady Memorial Hospital in Atlanta. This is where John Mooney was to do his residency and build his skills as a surgeon. When he entered the university as a young freshman, Emory had already enjoyed rather remarkable growth and expertise in most major areas of medicine—from treating all forms of viral and infectious diseases to the very latest in surgical procedures.

However, John wasn't only entering the world of medicine when he arrived on the Atlanta campus in the late summer of 1926. He was also entering a whole new social world, one in which he had very little experience coming from a small town and a very conservative family.

For example, the prohibitionist attitude he had about drinking as he was growing up and all through his high school years was soon to be challenged. However, he did manage to hang on to it through his freshman term. Spurred by the remnants of his low self-esteem, he plunged with great fervor into his studies, determined to launch his college career at the top of his class. And he did just that. He returned home to Statesboro pounding his chest with pride for being such a good student and such a good person. His family applauded him, although his younger sister did tease him a bit about being "a goodie two-shoes."

But all of that bravado only lasted until the week after his eighteenth birthday. While John returned to Emory University School of Medicine that summer to begin his sophomore year filled with positive intentions, he seemed unable for some reason to ignore all the other students around him having so much fun. They were joking and laughing. And they were drinking. It was the drinking that really caught his eye. He remembered as a youngster thinking that decent people didn't drink. Yet, his fellow students looked like very decent people. Sure, some of them were acting silly, but they seemed to be really enjoying themselves and each other's company.

Wherever he went over the next few weeks, he'd always seem to spot some people drinking—and having fun. Then one afternoon his roommate said he was going to a dance at the Allendale Country Club, not too far from school, and invited John to join him. He did. It was the early fall of 1928—and it turned out to be the night that completely changed his life.

That evening, his roommate and a group of frat guys he had befriended pulled him into a corner of the dance hall and began passing around an old tin can filled with corn liquor. When it came to John, he hesitated. It was either peer pressure or curiosity or his own natural instinct that made him put the can to his lips and take a big swallow. He started coughing . . . then took a second swallow to stop from choking. Everyone began to laugh as the corn liquor ran down his chin. As the young man next to him reached out for the tin can, John clutched it and put it back to his lips. For what John Mooney wanted at that moment was what he wanted all his life. He wanted more.

Some years later he would say, "As soon as that alcohol reached my brain, it put me off into another world. And I lived in that world for the next thirty years. In the beginning, I would come back into the real world to recuperate, to get things straightened out for a while. But when I was in the real world during those times, when I was off alcohol or drugs, I was always homesick for that other world. I used to think that it took a long time to become an alcoholic. That night it took me about one minute and forty-five seconds."

The doctor's son got very drunk that evening. He walked around in a blackout for a while until he finally passed out and his friends had to carry him back to the campus and dump him into his bed. He woke up the next morning with a terrible hangover and swore he would never do such a stupid thing again. And he didn't—for almost a month.

John discovered that it was easier to drink at fraternity parties. So before his senior year, he found himself a member of Sigma Chi, Alpha Kappa Kappa, and Omicron Delta Kappa. He patted himself on the back for achieving such a feat—membership in three elite fraternities. He gave little thought to the fact that he achieved it mostly because he wanted to drink and this gave him ample opportunity to get to the trough whenever he wished.

"I don't think anyone back then recognized alcoholism as a disease and a progressive disease at that," John would tell sober colleagues later on. "But I certainly began to slowly deteriorate, first in my scholarship. I stood fairly close to the top of my class when I started medical school but I began to drift down. By the time I finished, I wasn't anywhere near the top.

"But I didn't seem to let it bother me. I was beginning to suffer from an insidious disease without knowing it. My life began to revolve around alcohol more and more and when I wasn't actually drinking, I was thinking about it."

The young medical student quickly came to realize, however, that he couldn't drink as much as he might want to and still study and pass his exams. He couldn't let drinking interfere with or control his life. He had to be in control. So he laid out a plan for himself. While he was going through medical school, he wouldn't drink during exam periods or when studying for them. He would drink only when the examinations were over so he could celebrate a little. He would certainly not drink whenever he needed to drive anywhere, and he would try not to drink when home on vacation. And when he took up his residency in surgery, he would be especially careful never to get drunk. Once he felt comfortable that he had thought it all through, he went to one of his fraternity houses for another drink.

The truth is, John actually did stick pretty much to his plan. He would have serious drinking bouts from time to time, but being young and healthy, he did manage to control his appetite for liquor through most of his academic career. In fact, in his fourth year at Emory, he was elected class president. An accomplished violinist, he was also concertmaster in the school's respected symphony orchestra.

When he first started drinking, John never gave a thought to where his friends obtained their alcohol. But one day it struck him. This was the time of Prohibition. When the Eighteenth Amendment, or the Volstead Act, went into effect on January 16, 1920, all breweries, distilleries, and saloons were forced to close their doors. The Women's Christian Temperance Union had won the day and now America was to be a dry land—legally speaking, that is.

Certainly John had heard about speakeasies and such, but not in Statesboro. Then he realized how naive he was—that if people wanted to drink, they could probably find booze anywhere, even in his hometown. The more he thought about it, the more his thirst grew for another drink. So he inquired among his friends and learned they were buying their corn liquor from a bootlegger who made the stuff in the Okeefenokee Swamp. He was shocked when he realized the swamp area wasn't all that far from Statesboro.

Georgians had been making all kinds of bootleg liquor, better known as "Georgia moonshine," since the late 1800s. When Prohibition came along, it forced producers to move their operations deep into the state's rugged mountains and swamps, but it also turned their output into a very valuable and much sought-after commodity.

The distillation of apples, corn, or peaches into whiskey, brandy, or other forms of alcohol quickly became a cottage industry. The rapid expansion of the moonshine business also helped farmers across the state earn extra cash from supplying the illegal stills. This cash, in turn, enabled the farmers to increase their output of fruits and vegetables as well as cotton and tobacco, thus boosting the state's overall economy.

While the actual production of good moonshine liquor is quite an involved process, it's not so difficult that a whole generation of Georgia mountain men weren't able to master it. They did . . . learning how fermentation works, the careful mixture of the starches in the grain or fruit with sugar, yeast, and malt . . . the distillation process that creates the spirits of the alcohol . . . and the collection in jars, jugs, and other containers.

The biggest problem was distribution, especially when the federal government began to enforce the Prohibition law. FBI and Treasury agents flooded the countryside to chop down stills and arrest all the moonshiners they could round up. Also, Georgia's rugged terrain and poor roads at the time made delivery to eager customers all that more difficult.

So, it wasn't long before John Mooney helped solve that problem for himself and for his campus buddies. Through a friend, he met two men who made Georgia moonshine in the Ogeechee River Swamp. They worked out a deal. Soon they were loading up his car and he'd haul the stuff to Atlanta, where he would share it with his fellow students.

"I was accused one day by someone on campus of being a bootlegger," he joked with a friend later in life. "I felt indignant, them charging me with being a common moonshiner. I didn't say it then, but I'd like to set the record straight now. I didn't consider myself a bootlegger. I was merely selling the stuff for what it cost me . . . with just a slight handling charge, of course."

In 1929, the stock market crashed, ushering in the Great Depression. It affected practically everyone in America. Some of John's close friends at Emory were forced to leave school because neither they nor their parents could afford to pay the tuition or other costs related to the study of medicine. John was fortunate. Even though his father lost a substantial amount of money in the stock market, his other investments and his savings were still considerable. So he continued to pay for his son's education and his son was deeply grateful.

By 1933, however, the nation's financial crisis began to close in on the Mooney family. The economic depression was deepening. Industries, farmers, and the ordinary workingmen and -women had less money to spend or invest. It started to affect banks all across the country. They began to fail at an alarming rate.

In fact, it's estimated that more than four thousand banks closed their doors during 1933. Back then, there was no such thing as federal deposit insurance. If a bank failed, you simply lost all the money you had in that bank. Depositors are said to have lost more than $140 billion in 1933 alone.

The economic catastrophe that hovered over the nation for more than ten years didn't miss Statesboro or Dr. Mooney or the Bank of Statesboro that he and his friends owned. However, while other banks in the city shut their doors, leaving their depositors to frantically watch their hard-earned and much-needed funds disappear, Dr. Mooney refused to do the same. Instead, he bought out his shaken partners. Then he paid each and every one of his bank's depositors with his own money.

This somewhat heroic decision left the doctor almost broke. It took him many years to rebuild his estate. But his actions and his kindness to the citizens of the hard-hit city that day enhanced the reputation of the Mooney family far beyond the cost involved. And it would carry over to Dr. John Mooney Jr. when he set up his own practice in Statesboro.

After graduating from medical school, the new Dr. Mooney returned to Statesboro to support his father during this stressful time in his life. John had just been accepted as a surgical resident at Grady Hospital, which was now part of Emory University School of Medicine. He had also quietly approached several of Atlanta's remaining banks for a loan that would see him through for the next two years at Grady. He was greeted with looks of disbelief and quickly turned down. One bank manager almost laughed in his face.

When he suggested to his father that he might take a sabbatical for the next year or two, Dr. Mooney Sr. would not hear of it. He said he would manage somehow . . . and that his son would have plenty of time to pay him back once he began practicing medicine.

So John went back to Atlanta and began to hone his skills as a surgeon. Even though he worked very long hours at the hospital, he did manage to socialize from time to time. On one of those occasions, a surgeon he had befriended at Grady invited him to dinner at a country club on the outskirts of the city. He discovered that his doctor friend knew many people there, including a still rather wealthy attorney by the name of John S. Spaulding. The attorney was having dinner with his wife, Sarah, and their daughter, Sally Christian, a charming twenty-three-year-old debutante who seemed to sparkle as John was being introduced to her father. Before the evening was over, John and Sally Christian danced many dances together. He even wound up with a date to meet her at her home two weeks hence. As he was to comment some years later with a wide smile on his face, "She seemed to be the ideal girl for a man who was going to be a distinguished doctor, a man who was really going to wake up the whole world of medicine in the state of Georgia. They were going to know about me all right and admire my skills. So I needed to pick my wife very carefully because we wanted to move in the proper social circles, particularly somebody like me who was going to have all of this prestige, all this income, all of these summer and winter homes and fancy cars. I mean, all of this goes together with the proper breeding and culture, right? So I got married."

Little did John know that Sally Christian was thinking along the same lines: how wonderful it would be to be the wife of a famous surgeon, to throw big parties, to have people thanking you for your husband's saving their lives. If someone was paying close attention at the time, it would have sounded like this relationship was shaping up to be more like a partnership built on profit and prestige rather than one based on love and commitment. As you would expect, it turned out to be a big wedding. A real big wedding.

John and Sally Christian were married on October 17, 1935, while he was still doing his internship in general surgery at Grady Hospital. He was twenty-five and she had just turned twenty-four.

The wedding was what the society pages of the *Atlanta Constitution* described as "a brilliant ceremony for a brilliant couple" at St. Mark Methodist Church on Peachtree Street. The society pages went on to report that "rows of candelabra with tapered almond candles were festooned on the altar while white dahlias with white satin bows marked the pews reserved for the many prominent Georgia families in attendance."

Sally's sister, Miss Elizabeth Spaulding, was her maid of honor while John's best friend, Dr. William S. Mitchell, served as his best man. There were seven bridesmaids and seven groomsmen rounding out what the society pages concluded to be "one of the most elegant weddings ever to be held at old St. Mark Church." The extravagant indoor-outdoor wedding reception was held at the Spaulding estate on River Road in Atlanta. The wedding guests, many of whom came from other parts of the country, were treated to a lavish meal that concluded with a four-tier wedding cake.

Unless you read the newspapers that day, you would have never known that, while the wedding guests were dining at the Spaulding estate, there were millions of people elsewhere standing on soup lines or selling apples to feed their families.

Because of his demanding residency at Grady Hospital, the bride and groom had a brief honeymoon at an undisclosed location and then hurried back to Atlanta. Sally kept insisting that her father's connection at Emory could extend their stay. She started a small tiff when John refused the offer and an even bigger tiff over his bringing liquor with him and drinking too much. But they made up on the train ride home.

The following year John was named the assistant resident of surgery at Grady, which by now was a large and bustling hospital with a very busy emergency room. He would often have to work around the clock. He had a natural gift for surgery and was learning new surgical procedures almost every day. He loved it. Sally Christian hated it. She wanted him home with her and didn't believe he needed to work such long hours. When he did come home, he would sneak a few drinks just to withstand her constant complaining. The only thing that would stop her was the promises he would make about the wonderful future that lay ahead for them.

Finally, in the summer of 1938, Doctor John Mooney Jr. received his license to practice general surgery. While Sally knew about her husband's commitment to his father, that he would return to Statesboro and practice medicine out of his office, she still tried to persuade him to stay in Atlanta. She said there were many, many more patients in the large metropolitan city, a lot more money to be made, and between that and her father's connections, he could be a great success in no time. Rather than argue, her husband promised that if she really didn't like Statesboro after living there for a few years, he would seriously consider moving back to Atlanta. She went along with him, believing she would eventually get her way.

CHAPTER THREE

A Heroic Surgeon at War

YOUNG DR. JOHN MOONEY WAS DELIGHTED TO BE SETTING UP his medical practice in Statesboro, Georgia. He felt even more pleased knowing he was not only repaying the debt he owed his father for all his support through medical school but also because he'd be practicing in the building his father owned and where he had treated patients for so many years. It was something he dreamed about as a young boy.

The son of Dr. Alfonso John Mooney was returning home a skilled surgeon ready to practice that skill from the very day he arrived. Since he became so busy so quickly, his wife offered to help furnish his new office. She also wanted to feel like she was part of her doctor's life, not just someone who sat around looking pretty. But her serious lack of knowledge about medical procedures, the type of equipment and furnishings required, plus her short temper, led to frequent arguments. So she focused on the plans for their new home instead.

John had saved some money from his work at Grady Hospital. With that and a mortgage from his father's bank, he purchased an acre and a half of property on Lee Street and hired an architect to design a home for them. Not only was he excited about the project, but it also gave his wife something to do to keep her busy and out of his office.

The most important thing the surgeon had promised himself now that he was back in Statesboro was that he would quit drinking. Good doctors don't drink, he kept telling himself, and he wanted to be a good doctor. The best. That's why I can't drink and practice medicine, he told himself, particularly surgery. You have to be careful when dealing with human lives. So he stopped drinking. It lasted for about two weeks.

In one of his many talks some years later, he explained with tongue in cheek, "I found out the tensions of private practice were much greater than those of an internship. You learn in the medical field that tension can cause heart attacks and I was under a great deal of tension. I'd heard about doctors in their thirties and forties who worked themselves to death. They never got enough relaxation and died from heart attacks. I sure didn't want to do that. And I knew that a few drinks gave me a whole lot of relaxation. So I only drank to help my practice along."

He remembered the drinking plan he had worked out while going through medical school and tried to apply it to his medical practice. He didn't drink while treating patients and certainly not before surgery. He only drank when his day's work was over and he always tried never to get too drunk. He was still young, determined, and afraid—afraid of what might happen if he ever lost control. So he worked at controlling his drinking.

The next few years flew by. Between building the Lee Street house, their jaunts to Atlanta to visit his wife's parents and friends, and being the busiest surgeon in south Georgia, there wasn't much time for what you might call real togetherness. Add to that Sally's continued nagging about John's drinking every night when he'd come home later and later from the office or the hospital, and his feeble defense that a few drinks relieved the stress and tension of his work. It all added up to a serious strain on their relationship. Their marriage might have come apart right then and there had it not been for one of the greatest tragedies ever to hit America.

All of Statesboro was shocked when the news came across the radio that Sunday afternoon, December 7, 1941. The Japanese had attacked Pearl Harbor. More than three thousand Americans were killed and almost as many wounded. The following day, President Franklin Delano Roosevelt appeared before a joint session of Congress and declared, "Yesterday, December 7, 1941—a date which will live in infamy—the United States of America was suddenly and deliberately attacked by naval and air forces of the Empire of Japan."

The president then asked Congress to approve a resolution recognizing that a state of war existed between the United States and Japan. The vote to approve was loud, raucous, and unanimous. Three days later, Germany and Italy declared war against the United States, and America responded in kind. Dr. John Mooney Jr. was one of the first men in Statesboro to sign up for "the war that was to end all wars."

Sally thought it was wonderful to be sending her man off to battle. She had probably been looking for something to bolster her own ego at this point since being a doctor's wife was wearing thin—particularly the wife of a drinking doctor. Now she could hang a star in her window and brag to all her friends at the bridge club how her heroic hubby would be saving the lives of all those brave soldiers on the battlefield.

She stayed in Statesboro during the first two years of the war. Then, to the surprise of many of her friends, she decided to close up the house and move back to Atlanta to live with her parents. She came back shortly before her husband returned home.

John's parents, sisters, and his many good friends in town, recognizing the nature and character of the man, knew that he had to go, but they weren't all that happy about it. In fact, his father knew what his son would be up against as a medical surgeon at the front lines and he worried a great deal. So did his mother, who had tried so hard to protect him as a youth. Now she was helpless to do anything for him except pray. And pray she did.

Following enlistment, the young surgeon was immediately assigned to the Medical Corps of the U.S. Army's famous Eighty-Second Airborne Division and sent to Fort Benning, Georgia, for his initial military training. From there he was shipped to Fort Bragg, North Carolina, for parachute and glider-borne training. These were the invasion tactics that were to be used in upcoming battle campaigns. After completing his military training, John was named a captain in the Medical Corps.

His next and most important assignment was learning how to set up and operate a field hospital behind the front lines, one that would provide the necessary surgical services and care for the severely wounded. The Medical Corps knew that the field hospitals of World War I would no longer be effective since modern warfare had brought many changes to the battlefield. The old field hospitals took too long to build and were usually set up many miles behind the lines.

Captain Mooney was put in charge of what was now called a portable or a "mobile medical unit," one that was manned by skilled surgeons, nurses, and medics and located close to the fighting. It was similar to the "MASH" units used in the Korean War that were made famous by the television show of the same name. The portable unit was designed to be moved by its own personnel and able to render quick, lifesaving surgical intervention for the troops.

In addition to learning all about setting up mobile hospitals, it took Mooney time to accomplish two other difficult tasks: parachuting with full gear and hard landings in equipment-filled gliders. That's when he first started smoking cigarettes. He found they calmed his nerves. When his commanders felt he and his team were ready for combat, he was shipped overseas to face the enemy—and his smoking picked up even more.

John first saw action when he parachuted into North Africa

in the spring of 1943, landing on the outskirts of Casablanca. German resistance was light, but there were still a number of American casualties to be treated. It was a chance for the captain and his team to gain experience working together and to get ready for the bigger battles that lay ahead. They were soon to come. The Eighty-Second Airborne Division moved quickly into Tunisia, capturing the remaining German troops and readying itself for one of the largest combined Allied campaigns of the war—the invasion of Sicily.

On the night of July 9, 1943, Captain John Mooney joined more than 180,000 other soldiers, sailors, and airmen, parachuting with his medical team onto the rocky island at the "toe" of Italy's boot. The Germans and Italians were well dug in and the battle for Sicily raged on for thirty-eight days. When the Axis finally surrendered the island, more than 2,200 Americans lay dead with 6,500 wounded. The British lost some 3,000 troops and accounted for 2,700 wounded.

Captain Mooney and his surgical team saved many lives during that campaign, which was an important one. Sicily was the first piece of the Axis homeland that had now fallen to the Allied forces. Also, it served as a great training ground for the many officers, enlisted men, and Medical Corps personnel, who, eleven months later, would be landing on the beaches of Normandy. But when the last bullet of the Sicily campaign was finally fired, John needed a drink. He needed one very badly.

He and several of his fellow medics found their way into the town of Syracuse, which was now partly in ruins. But they managed to locate a small restaurant and a wooden case filled with Chianti wine, something John referred to as "Sicilian moonshine." It did the trick. It put him into that unreal world that he enjoyed so much. And in that unreal world he was no longer afraid. The fear he had lived with for thirty-eight long days of blood, guts, and the mangled bodies of heroic soldiers was gone. He now felt comfortable and courageous.

But the young lady who was serving them obviously didn't feel the same way. While she was quite attractive in her wrinkled dress and stained apron, John could see the terror on her face and in her eyes from all she had been through. He tried to put her at ease, to make her smile, to let her know he was not her enemy. Though their languages were different, their needs were the same. They needed to feel safe, even if it were just for the moment. So he stayed with her that night to comfort her. They made love.

It wasn't until the next morning, when John sobered up and was heading back to his unit that the guilt hit. He had been praying to his God every single night to keep him safe and close. Last night he didn't pray. He drank and fornicated. Sure, he could blame it on the fighting, the fear, the loneliness, and the anger over losing too many innocent, torn-apart young soldiers. Still, the guilt stayed with him for the rest of the war.

By 1944, the Germans had defeated France and Poland and essentially controlled all of Europe. They knew that the Allies would soon be attempting an invasion to liberate the Continent and that it would probably take place somewhere along the French coast. So they heavily fortified all the cliffs overlooking the English Channel with huge cannon, cement bunkers, and machine gun nests.

On June 6, 1944, American, British, Canadian, and Australian forces, under the command of General Dwight David Eisenhower, landed more than 200,000 troops on five beachheads stretching fifty miles along the Normandy peninsula. From the shore of the English Channel to the top of the French palisades, brave fighting men were met with fierce resistance. It was heroic doctors like Captain John Mooney who parachuted into the fray under fire and, even though wounded himself, helped set up the mobile hospitals that saved many thousands of lives over the ensuing days, weeks, and months that followed.

On D-Day alone, more than 6,000 American soldiers were

killed and almost 9,000 were wounded. By the end of the Normandy campaign, nearly 425,000 Allied and Axis troops were either killed or wounded, or were missing in action.

John's wound healed quickly. He stayed with his mobile hospital unit as it followed the Eighty-Second Airborne Division through bloody battles all across Europe. He managed to treat the mounting casualties despite some of the biggest hardships he and his team had to face, like food and drug shortages, and some of the worst rainy, icy, and snowy weather conditions imaginable. And there were always the other problems too—lack of sterile supplies, surgical drapes, sutures, and dressings, and even small things like leaky tents, lack of hot water, and no surgical soap. Too often when operating at night with the ground shaking from incoming shell fire and ack-ack guns, the hand-cranked generators would fail and the lights would go out in the middle of the procedure. Yet somehow Captain Mooney and his medical team would muddle through and perform real lifesaving miracles along the way.

At the same time, John was finding himself drinking more and more every time one battle would end and before another one would begin. He was trying hard to stick with the plan he had laid out for himself back home—not to drink when treating patients and certainly not when performing surgery. But it was getting more and more difficult to maintain his control. That's when he began using drugs.

It was during his last campaign of the war—the invasion of Holland on September 17, 1944. John was flying in a glider together with his surgical team and all the equipment they needed for their mobile hospital. They were due to land in an area near the Nijmegen-Groesbeek Bridge, which, in 1977, became the subject of a big movie called *A Bridge Too Far*. American forces had been holding off ferocious German counterattacks on the bridge, which resulted in significant casualties.

Many gliders had crashed during the war, killing many American troops when landing on rocks, or in trees, streams, and rivers.

As a result, they were cynically called "The Bastards No One Wanted." Tragically, John's glider crashed that night, seriously injuring many on board, including him. He came away with a back injury that limited his ability to handle his medical duties for a short time. But again, he got back into action quickly, only this time with the help of a drug called Demerol. He had found a new friend, one that wouldn't interfere with his work as alcohol did. At least that's what he thought at the start of their fond relationship.

In the spring of 1945, shortly after Germany had surrendered, John was shipped back to the States. A few days before he was to leave for home, he began sweating and shivering from a bad cold. Fearing it could turn into pneumonia, he checked into a nearby hospital, where the doctor promptly put him to bed and prescribed some medication. As the doctor was about to leave the room, John saw him turn to an attending nurse and whisper, "There lies a case of war nerves if I ever saw one."

Upon hearing what he considered to be a very sympathetic remark, the young, battle-weary physician responded rather loudly, "Hey, Doc. Just give me a shot of Demerol and I'll be fine."

Dr. John Mooney not only got his wish that day and the day after, but as he lay back in his hospital bed, he began to realize he had just been given something else even more important than a shot of Demerol. He was given something he could use to the fullest over the weeks and months ahead—"war nerves," an excuse to drink and take a few drugs without feeling the least bit of guilt.

So, while the young physician was no longer under enemy fire and his wounds and injuries had basically healed, he was coming home with an addict's best friend—an ailment most people would not only understand and tolerate but would also accept as a combat-related nervous condition. The heroic surgeon's "war nerves" would surely justify a few drinks now and then to keep things under control. When he finally arrived home, he found it worked like a charm, except, that is, with his unhappy and disillusioned wife, Sally Christian.

Captain John Mooney came home to a hero's welcome. He had received a Purple Heart, two Bronze Stars with Oak Leaf Clusters, a Presidential Citation, and a Distinguished Unit Award. He came home an alcoholic and drug addict who was totally in denial. He also came home to a wife he barely recognized, and who barely recognized him.

While most of the people in Statesboro put John on a pedestal, it seemed like Sally Christian could see right through him. He thought she would be excited to have him home. She was, at least for the first few weeks or so. Then reality set in as she watched him smoking too much and drinking too much at almost every party they attended, at every festivity thrown in his honor. He couldn't see why she didn't understand that he was simply treating his "war nerves," something he told her about in detail that first night home when he crawled into bed with her too drunk to make love. But that wasn't the only thing John couldn't see.

His vision of their life and his attitude toward it were poles apart from his wife's perceptions. He was blind to all the problems she was constantly laying out before him, problems she insisted were caused mainly by his drinking. He was merely unwinding from the war, he would proclaim, and all her constant nagging was creating even more reasons for him to unwind.

Some years later, when the physician's vision and attitude began to change, he would often tell the following story to illustrate where he was at this point in his marriage:

There are three young women who apply for jobs as airline hostesses. After going through all the written examinations, there is one oral test left. It has to do with a potential situational problem, one that would help determine what their attitude is toward men.

They are called in front of a panel of examiners one at a time. As the first young lady makes herself comfortable, one of the examiners proposes the following:

"We want you to imagine that you are a hostess on a transoceanic airliner. It has gotten into trouble and has to ditch in the middle of the ocean. You are the sole survivor and you find yourself adrift on a small life raft. As you float in the hot, burning sun, the days and nights grow longer and longer. You become terrified, filled with despair and figure there is no way out.

"Just when you're about to give up all hope, you look off into the distance and see what appears to be land. As you get still closer, you discover that it really is land. Your hope rises. You become filled with anticipation. Now you see that it is a lush and beautiful island. You become filled with jubilation—that is, until you discover that on the island are twenty-five U.S. marines that haven't seen a girl in over a year. What would you do?"

The first young lady hesitates for a moment, then blurts out that she would have no problem with the situation. She says the water around the island would have currents and that life rafts have paddles. She would simply paddle away and look for another island.

They call in the second girl, lay out the same scenario, and ask what she would do. She also says it would be no problem since she always has her handbag on her shoulder with a revolver inside. She concludes that the revolver would be adequate protection under the circumstances.

The examiners then call in the third young woman and almost before they've finished their remarks, she leans forward in her chair, smiles at them and says, "Gentlemen, I've heard the situation, but what's the problem?"

And that's how it was at this point with Dr. John Mooney. After all he had been through and the manner in which he had gotten through it, he just couldn't see the problem.

His war experience had honed John into an exceptional surgeon, and the people of Statesboro greatly admired him for his skill and heroics. Still, the young physician knew he was also living and succeeding partly off his father's much-heralded reputation in the community. The stories of his great generosity during the Depression and his enormous medical, business, and civic contributions over the years were now carved in stone.

All that became obviously clear once again when Dr. Alfonso John Mooney Sr. passed away on December 12, 1946, at the age of seventy-one. A pall settled over all of Statesboro during his funeral. That's how revered he was. And his death struck his son like the enemy bombardment on D-Day. John had all he could do to hold himself together and be strong for his mother and the family. Even though his father had been ill for some time with lung cancer, his passing still came as a painful shock. It always does when we don't want to lose someone we cherish.

As John stood next to the beautiful oak casket at the funeral parlor, he was filled with guilt and regret, remembering the day a few months back when his father, despite his weakened condition, came to his house because he heard his son hadn't been to work in almost a week. He found him lying in bed, drunk.

"I remember telling him I was sick," John admitted some years later. "But my father could smell the booze, and the look on his face made me feel deeply ashamed. I don't think I had ever felt so low before in my life."

The elderly doctor, who had been a teetotaler all his life, sat down beside the bed and, for the very first time, talked to his son about his drinking.

"I had a sense you were taking a few drinks now and then," John's father said, "but I never knew it had come to this. I know you and Sally are having some problems, but carrying on like this isn't going to make them any better, son. Promise me you will stop."

Still staring at his father's casket, John remembered promising his dad he would stop, then continuing to drink after he left. The young surgeon didn't see his father for several weeks before he passed away. He would carry that guilt with him for years—until he finally sobered up and found a way to make amends.

The surgeon sipped secretly from a flask throughout the funeral services and burial in the stately family plot. He waited a few days until his mother was settled back in her home with his sisters watching over her. Then he went on a real toot. And between his "war nerves" and his father's death, it was a dandy of a toot. He had to take a few days off from work to recover. Sally refused to clean up his mess.

Before John had gone off to war, he and Sally Christian were at least civil to each other most of the time and even a little loving every once in a while. But now, after his being home more than a year, she had become a cold and completely unhappy stranger. When they talked, she would want to know what he did during the war. Where was he? Who was he with? What were his nurses like? Were they pretty? Why didn't he write more? And then there was always his drinking. She wouldn't let up. Between her suspicions of him while he was overseas and her screaming tantrums about his boozing at home, he decided it couldn't go on like this. It had to come to a head one way or the other.

As an old friend remembers it, John decided they had to either try to make a new start or end the marriage once and for all. In order to make a new start, he insisted they both be totally open and honest with each other about the four years when they were apart. So, after drinking quite a bit, John told his wife about the hardships of war, his anger over losing young soldiers on the operating table, even some funny but embarrassing moments at their mobile hospital unit. Then, after a slight nervous hesitation, he told her about his brief affair with a young woman in Italy, whom he never really knew except for that one night. The very next day, Sally Christian Spaulding Mooney packed up and moved back to Atlanta, where she filed for divorce on the grounds of infidelity.

John didn't fight it. Instead, he got drunk again. He got very drunk. And he stayed drunk until one day, in between his terrible hangovers, he came to realize that you can't be a recognized, prestigious, and very wealthy physician if you're drunk all the time. So, using every ounce of willpower and self-control he could muster, he got sober one more time and threw himself into his work. He built more than a respectable practice and began making a whole lot of money. Dr. John Mooney Jr. had no other interests in his life at that point except the practice of medicine—that is, until Dorothy Carolyn Riggs came along.

CHAPTER FOUR

A Real Country Gal

"PEOPLE WHO HAVE NEVER LIVED IN THE COUNTRY—I MEAN, the real country—I believe are underprivileged."

That's what the pert, pretty and party-loving gal named Dorothy Carolyn Riggs, the daughter of a farming family from Jimps, Georgia, used to say with a big smile to friends and strangers alike because she really and truly meant it.

"I grew up in the country, swimming in ponds and rivers, swinging from tree limbs, fishing for catfish with my older brother, Arthur James, and filling baskets with wild berries as we tramped through the woods. Then we'd stuff ourselves with newly harvested corn, turnips, and watermelon and wash it all down with fresh milk or apple cider. I've always felt kind of sorry," she would conclude, "that there are people who have never had the opportunity to grow up and be part of country life. I loved it."

Dorothy Carolyn Riggs, who was known as "Dot" to all her friends and neighbors, was proud of the fact that she came from the small rural community of Jimps, located on Highway 301 about five miles down the road from Statesboro, Georgia. She was born in her family's farmhouse on October 23, 1922.

Back then, everything in Jimps centered on the railroad. In town, people lived in houses that stood on both sides of the tracks, unless you lived on one of the many family farms in the area. There were two general stores that stood across from one another on a dirt road near the small railroad station. One of them was owned by Dot's father, Arthur Riggs, who also had a cotton gin right behind the store and a small family farm nearby. There was also a dress shop in town, a small restaurant, and the post office, among a few other enterprises.

For its size, Jimps was very much a thriving social and commercial center in the early days of Bulloch County—that is, until the late 1920s, when the boll weevil came to Georgia and began to devastate all the cotton fields, including those in Jimps and the surrounding area. That and the stock market crash of 1929, which sparked the Great Depression, slowly began to impact the lives of everyone in this small town.

While those ominous shadows were looming on the horizon, they didn't really affect Dot's early growing-up years. She came from a very secure home, although it was one with little or no outward signs of affection. As she would say later on, while she knew she was loved, neither her mother, Myrtis, nor her father, Arthur, ever told her so. And she wanted someone to tell her. She wanted to hear it, to feel it, and she never really did—not until she met John Mooney Jr.

There were four children in the Riggs family, two younger twin sisters, Dot, and her older brother, Arthur James, who worked the farm with his father. And because she was the older daughter, much of the responsibility for cleaning, washing, and other chores fell on her shoulders. She didn't mind it too much until she became a teenager and wanted to have more freedom and more fun, which wasn't all that unusual for teenagers. But it began to create real conflict with her mother, who was a strict disciplinarian.

Myrtis was also a strict taskmaster when it came to her religion. Her daughter once said her mother used to brag that the first place she took her was to church. Dot was three weeks old at the time and later felt that, because she was at church so often, she was raised in one of the pews. Her mother used to describe herself as "a Godfearing woman."

"Maybe that's why I grew up with this terrible fear of God," Dot would share later on in her life, "listening to all this fire and brimstone stuff and that you were going right to Hell if you do something wrong. I wish my mother had called herself a 'God-loving' woman instead and maybe I wouldn't have had so much fear. It took me years to find a loving God and to lose all that fear."

Despite all of that, the young girl wasn't really Cinderella with a witch for a mother. She had many fond memories of her growing-up years—swimming in the nearby pond and the river and the creek when they would swell after a heavy rain. She was very close to her brother. He included her in almost everything he did, even playing with him and the boys in his crowd.

Dot once said, "Whatever my brother and those other boys did, I did too. Maybe that's why I came to love men so much. I don't have any problems with women, but I just love men. I appreciate them. And I think it's because I did have an older brother who I dearly loved and was part of his crowd and everything they did."

So, growing up, even with all the chores she had to handle, Dot's life was filled with fun and excitement. She enjoyed riding saddle horses on the weekends and when her father would let her handle the mules as they plowed the fields to plant cotton and corn and watermelons and other crops. She even enjoyed those mornings in the chicken houses, listening to the hens cluck as she helped gather the eggs that her father sold at his general store. As she often said, she loved being a country gal.

Her dad was a hardworking man but soft and easygoing, and a man who drank too much once in a while. But so did her mother, who, unlike her father, was a strong and dominating woman. Before marrying Arthur, she had led a sad and lonely life. Deserted by her father at age thirteen, she and her mother had to make it by themselves and it was a struggle. Hard work and drive were what sustained them and were probably what turned Myrtis into something her children called "a slave driver." Nothing was ever good enough, and nothing was ever done right unless it was done her way.

Young Dot also didn't like the way her mother treated her husband. She was often very harsh and picked arguments with him over nothing. Dot loved her dad very much. One night, as a young teenager, she walked out onto the front porch of their farmhouse to find her father sitting in his favorite rocker, smoking his pipe. He looked tired and sad. She knelt down next to him with tears running down her cheeks and said she couldn't stand living in the same house with her mother any longer and was going to leave. He kept on rocking for a moment, then stopped, looked at her, and said, "Honey, I understand what you're saying because I can't hardly live with her myself, but I got nowhere to go. We all got to do what we got to do."

As she hugged her father, she realized she couldn't leave him. She loved him too much. So she stayed there and took care of him until she finished high school. And in the meantime, she tried to have as much fun as she could at every opportunity she could find.

The pert and pretty teenager was very popular with all the kids at her local high school, boys and girls alike. And she enjoyed being with them at school functions as well as barn dances and house parties. After some maneuvering, she finally got her mother's permission to invite a group of her high school friends to her own house.

The truth was, Myrtis had always regretted being deprived of normal teen fun in her own life and was now afraid that if she didn't ease up on her domineering ways, her daughter might just pack up and run off. So Dot now began using any excuse at all to invite a gang of her friends to her farmhouse for a party. They'd move back the furniture in the parlor, roll up the rug, and dance for hours to records she played on the new Victrola her father had bought for the family. As the young teenager remembered that time in her life with some nostalgia, she said it was sort of her innocent, coming-of-age period and one that fueled her desire to keep on partying.

It was also around this time that Dot got her license to drive. One balmy summer day, she drove out to the home of some cousins who lived near a lake not many miles away. She planned to spend a week's vacation with them. A few days after her arrival, her young relatives threw a welcoming party for her. That's where Dot had her first magical experience with alcohol.

She remembered the churning in her stomach that night, the throwing up, and the pounding headache the next morning. But what the teenager remembered most of all was the thrill of flying through the great, blue Carolina skies that afternoon and the contentment that comes from being so happily at peace with the world and everyone in it. There was also the freedom that springs from the belief that you are important, admired, and respected. What she didn't understand then and for a long time afterward is that alcohol lies to you. It deceives, destroys, and ultimately takes everything that is precious in your life. Dorothy Carolyn Riggs was to be no exception.

While the teenager was enjoying her newfound freedom, she was also well aware of what was going on around her—the growing effects of the nation's economic depression on her family and the many people in town and throughout the area. At the same time, the boll weevil was continuing to wipe out more and more cotton farms in south Georgia, including those in Jimps and Statesboro. As a result, Dot's father had to shut down his cotton gin due to the lack of business.

With less cash in their pockets, many people began bartering for goods and services—a chicken for the doctor's fee, eggs for gas, a radio for a month's rent. Some families like the Riggs were more fortunate because they had a working farm where they grew their own food and raised their own cows and hogs and chickens. They were not only able to feed themselves but could also sell or share their excess with their neighbors and friends.

Still, for many in the state of Georgia, the depression was a catastrophe. Bank failures were common, and in small towns and communities, opportunities for loans dried up. Small businesses such as Arthur Riggs's general store were especially vulnerable. Less money in circulation meant fewer paying customers. With the absence of credit and financing, many business owners quickly went under. However, because he had his farm to fall back on, the Riggs family managed to survive the worst of the economic storm.

It was 1939. Dot had just turned seventeen and was getting bored simply helping out around the house and the farm. She had hoped to find a little job in town or possibly in nearby Statesboro, but there were none to be had. And her relationship with her mother was deteriorating once again to where they were now constantly at each other. Then one day a thought came to her—wouldn't it be nice to be a nurse and help people in need. She had always been willing to do that, but where the idea of nursing came from she never really knew. Suddenly, however, she was convinced that nursing was to be her calling, her vocation.

Surprisingly, her mother agreed. In fact, she seemed quite pleased with her daughter's decision. She even helped her find a nursing school she could apply to that was not all that far away. While Myrtis was happy her daughter wanted to be a nurse, she still didn't want her to be too far from home.

The closest one they could locate was the Warren A. Candler School of Nursing in Savannah. It just happened to be one of the finest nursing schools in the state. It was also part of Candler Hospital, the first hospital established in Georgia back in 1804 and the second-oldest continuously operating hospital in the United

States. So, Dorothy Riggs applied, and because of her excellent grades throughout high school, she was immediately accepted.

Despite her problems with her mother, the young and still very immature country gal began to miss her father, her brother, her sisters, and all her friends back in Jimps more than she realized. She thought what she wanted was total freedom, to stand on her own two feet, to be Miss Independence. But instead, she was getting homesick. Savannah was too far away. She managed to last almost two years at Warren A. Candler. She became so lonely that she began having occasional fits of panic and nervous spells. She finally decided to leave and return home.

By now it was wartime. The Japanese had attacked Pearl Harbor. Many of the young men she knew in town, including her brother, whom she adored, were being called into service to fight the Germans and the Italians in Europe and the Japanese in the South Pacific. Women were joining the WACS (Women's Army Corps) and the WAVES (Women Accepted for Volunteer Emergency Service, the women's branch of the U.S. Naval Reserve), and nurses were enlisting to care for the war wounded. Suddenly there was a serious nursing shortage here at home.

One day Dot received a phone call from the administrator of Bulloch County Hospital in Statesboro. He said he had her records from Warren A. Candler and wanted to know if she was still interested in nursing. When Dot replied that she was, the administrator immediately offered her a job as what he termed "a practical nurse," and at a very decent salary. She was ecstatic and quickly accepted the offer. And she wasn't the least bit nervous about it because she'd be working in Statesboro, a town not all that far from Jimps and her family.

Recalling those exciting yet anxious times back in the early 1940s, Dot would say, "I felt this was my chance to help out with the war effort. I went to work at the hospital and before long I was doing all the things the other nurses did. Between the training I had received at Warren Candler in Savannah and what I was being taught by the Bulloch County Hospital staff, I became a very good nurse. And I really loved nursing.

"I know I should have finished my training, but, looking back, I was still very young at the time and very immature. I used to worry about it until I came to understand that it was meant to be just the way it was. If I had finished nursing school in Savannah, my life may not have ended up like it did. And I wouldn't change anything in my life—all the disappointments, the frustrations, the heartache, and the shame—because in the end, it turned out to be too good for me to want it any other way."

So the young lady from the country moved into the city and found a small apartment for rent in an older woman's home. She began to make friends very quickly. Soon she was being invited to parties where there was lots of drinking. She was only slightly taken aback at first by all the liquor around her because she hadn't drunk that much after her first bout with alcohol at her cousins' house. And at school in Savannah, she only had a few drinks on weekends because she was always fearful of coming back to her dorm room "too tipsy" and then being too hung over to make her classes.

But now it was a different story. She was really on her own and could come and go as she pleased. And even though she began putting in long hours at the hospital right from the start, she became willing and eager to join her fellow nurses and staffers for a few drinks after work—and it was often more than just a few drinks.

Soon she was open to partying not only with her friends at the hospital but also with the many new companions she was getting to meet in Statesboro's social circle. In no time at all, Dot Riggs got to know practically every girl in town who enjoyed drinking, so she was never without companionship. She particularly enjoyed going out dancing, and the young nurse could dance to the swing music of the big bands for hours on end.

There happened to be an army training base not many miles

away, and soon Statesboro became one of the hundreds of small communities all over the country to open its doors to our fighting men. They would fill the club on West Main Street every weekend, and Dot got to meet them all. As she once recalled, "Since I knew so many girls who loved to party, I sort of played master of ceremonies every weekend when a bunch of soldiers would be coming to town. I'd make a few phone calls and I'd get ten to fifteen girls to show up at the club. The soldiers would bring the liquor and we gals would bring the food and we'd party and dance all night. I loved it and thought I was having the time of my life."

Perhaps it was the wartime, the shortage of skilled personnel, and the desire to keep everyone happy that slackened the rules at Bulloch County Hospital. Dot and many of her coworkers would have a drink now and then while still on duty and think nothing of it. None of the supervisors would bat an eye, and quite often they would also imbibe.

At the same time, the young practical nurse tried to make sure that her drinking never interfered with her work because she really enjoyed caring for her patients. There was an older gentleman patient she became particularly friendly with at the time. He was recovering from a serious automobile accident that resulted from his driving under the influence of alcohol. While very drunk, he ran his car off the road and into a tree. He was in traction with a broken leg and several other broken bones.

Dot discovered his buddies were bringing him bottles of booze and stashing them in the small metal cabinet next to his bed so they could be within his reach. One afternoon she entered his room unexpectedly to find him nipping out of one of the liquor bottles. He invited her to have a drink with him. She did, and before long it became a regular routine. As she explained very glibly once to some of her friends, "I had been taught as a nurse to do everything you can to make your patient comfortable and happy. So I would have a drink or two with him when I would get off work each afternoon. Actually it was probably more than a drink or two because I would sometimes sit there and talk with him for two or three hours.

"The truth is, I saw absolutely nothing wrong with it. There was nothing in our hospital's policies that said you couldn't go into a patient's room and sit down and have a few drinks with him. It never occurred to me there was anything wrong about it. In fact, I never worried about being caught doing it because it seemed to help the patient—and it also helped me."

The young nurse's relationship with her alcoholic patient came in handy one weekend when she was out partying with her girl-friends and some soldiers. They ran out of liquor and one of the soldiers suggested they go visit a bootlegger he knew on the out-skirts of Statesboro. Now Dot had heard her parents often talk about bootleggers and that young ladies should never go near them or else they could get into serious trouble. That's when she thought about her patient and all the liquor he had stashed in his metal cabinet.

So she talked her friends into driving her to the hospital, prom-ising them an ample supply of booze in return. It was about two o'clock in the morning when they arrived at Bulloch County Hos-pital and Dot was already quite intoxicated. She entered through the back door and managed to stagger into the man's room, al-most tripping in her high heels. She woke him up and asked if she could borrow a bottle of his liquor and said that she would pay him back when she got the money. He said she had taken such good care of him that she could have all she wanted for nothing.

The prettily dressed practical nurse took a fifth of rye whiskey from his cabinet and thanked him profusely. Only now she faced another dilemma. How does she get the booze out of the hospital? She had forgotten to bring her purse to put it in and you can't just stroll down a hospital corridor openly carrying a bottle of whis-key in your arms. Suddenly, despite her rather inebriated state, she found the answer. She'd carry it out in a bedpan.

She had been slinging bedpans around at the hospital long

enough to know that no one would stop and ask what's in it. So she took the large, enamel bedpan out from beneath her patient's cabinet and poured the fifth of rye into it. Then she slipped the bedpan into the white paper sack she always used to cover it, thanked the man once again, and staggered out of the hospital to continue partying.

When the young country gal awoke the next morning with a terrible hangover and remembered carrying booze in a bedpan, she felt quite embarrassed. Then she realized she had been doing more and more crazy things like that of late, and she wasn't happy about it at all. Deep inside she knew that alcohol was playing too big a role in her life and that maybe she should find other things to do aside from drinking and partying all the time.

Dorothy Carolyn Riggs was no longer going to church. She had stopped worshipping God each Sunday ever since she left for nursing school in Savannah. Despite many arguments with her mother about it when she returned home, she still never went back. And she was rarely praying anymore. Maybe that's the reason why, she thought to herself, her principles, which she always held high, were beginning to slip. She also remembered something she had said to one of her nondrinking colleagues at the hospital who had invited Dot to join her church.

"I respect people who attend church, but I won't lie to you about the way I feel," she told the woman. "I plan on having all the fun I want to and do all the living I want to and then when I'm too old to do anything else, I'll join a church."

As she sat on the edge of her bed that morning pondering the things she was doing while under the influence of alcohol, things she never intended to do, she soon found herself trying to justify her actions. She hadn't learned yet, since that first bout with booze at her cousins' place, that alcohol lies to you—makes you blame other people and happenstance, helps you to become a perfectionist in the art of self-deception.

While she enjoyed drinking and dancing and having a whole lot of fun, she told herself, she wasn't really running around with every Tom, Dick, and Harry like some other girls were doing. She wasn't going out with other people's husbands or becoming a loose woman with a bad reputation. She knew her friends and coworkers respected her and saw her as just a young woman who really enjoyed life. And her reputation was very important to her.

Still, Dot loved it when her friends would tell her how great it was she could drink all night and then get up and go to work the next morning. Her recuperative powers really were quite impressive. Yet, she knew her heavy drinking couldn't go on indefinitely. She was partying at a frenzied pace and her hangovers were getting worse. More important, she was beginning to have some difficulty functioning at top form at the hospital. So she tried to cut back on her drinking, but without much success.

It was now 1946. The war with Germany and Japan had ended, and our heroic fighting men were returning home in droves. Statesboro for a while became one big cabaret of celebration—parades, parties, and all-night bashes. And Dot found herself in the midst of it all.

One day at the hospital, after she had experienced a rather wild night of drinking followed by very little sleep, a fellow nurse joined her at the always-present coffeepot. After some small talk and commiseration over their long, hard hours of work, her friend asked if she had heard about the new diet pills called amphetamines that everyone was talking about. She said they kept you awake and alert after a night of partying and also helped with your weight, which had always been one of Dot's concerns.

It didn't take long for the young nurse to find a friendly doctor who wrote her a prescription for the pills. Now suddenly, she could do it all. What a marvelous invention. She could drink and dance and work, all without one thing causing any conflict with the other. Or so she thought. Again, Dot didn't know that drugs also lie to you just as alcohol does. She also didn't know that her real descent was about to begin. Soon she would need new and more powerful drugs to help her live the life she thought she enjoyed living.

She was first introduced to some of those powerful drugs when she faked having an appendicitis attack. She explained the rather bizarre decision some years later when sharing her experiences with a large group of recovered alcoholics and drug addicts: "I was getting tired and worn out from working so hard at the hospital and going out almost every night. I had already used up all my vacation and sick time, so I had to figure out a way to get some rest. Being a rather creative person, I decided to get appendicitis. This way when they operated, I would be in a comfortable hospital bed for at least three or four weeks.

"I knew how to run my temperature up, and I knew where it was supposed to hurt. Being a nurse, I knew a lot about the symptoms you're supposed to have. So they performed an appendectomy on me and after the surgery, they gave me Demerol and codeine, two powerful drugs that were to eventually become my constant companions. I still remember lying in that bed recuperating and just floating about halfway between the bed and the ceiling. I remember the first time I had that feeling as a teenager. I liked it. I hated the addiction part, but I love that feeling."

Fate was now about to step in and change Dot's life in a way she could have never dreamed. It all began when her landlady notified her she would have to find another place to live. She said her daughter had completed college, married her college sweetheart, was returning to Statesboro, and would need the apartment.

Again, as fate would have it, the young nurse had gotten to know a lady by the name of Mrs. Sally Christian Mooney. Dot would see Mrs. Mooney occasionally at the hospital when she dropped by to visit with her husband, Dr. John Mooney Jr., who had recently returned from the war. All she knew about Dr. Mooney was from rumors that he drank too much once in a while, but that he was loved and respected by practically everyone in Statesboro.

Dot bumped into Sally one day at a local store and, during a brief conversation, mentioned for some reason that she had lost her apartment and was looking for a new place to live. Mrs. Mooney quickly offered her the upstairs room in their comfortable home on Lee Street. She said she had been renting it to an elderly college professor who had recently retired and moved out. It couldn't be more perfect for the young nurse, since it was within walking distance of the hospital. So she took it.

After Dot moved in, she discovered that Sally and her husband were rarely home, so contact between them was practically nonexistent. Then one day, shortly after she had returned from work, she was surprised when Dr. Mooney knocked on her door. He explained to her quite unemotionally that he and his wife were getting a divorce. He wanted her to know because, in those days, it would not have been considered proper or acceptable for a young lady to rent a room from a bachelor, which Dr. Mooney was about to become.

As it turned out, Dot also knew Honey Bowen, who lived with her husband, Bill Bowen, just a few houses away. Bill was the mayor of Statesboro and owned a large furniture store in the city and a big farm in the country. Honey Bowen more or less headed the city's social set, although she was very much a down-to-earth person and a charming and caring woman with little or no phoniness about her. The same was true of her husband. So, when Honey heard of the Mooneys' mess—they had all been good friends—and Dot's plight, she rented the nurse one of the rooms in her large home until she could find a more accommodating place to live.

For some reason, the young nurse couldn't get Dr. Mooney off her mind. That sad look on his handsome face and the melancholy sound in his voice the day he knocked on her door to tell her about his divorce kept haunting her. When he was making his rounds at the hospital, she would go out of her way just to observe him, to notice the way he was admired by the staff, how highly regarded he was as a surgeon, how he seemed to stand ten feet tall over all the over physicians. She tried to deny it, but she was developing a crush on the man, even though he was thirteen years her senior.

One day coming out of a patient's room, Dot ran headlong into John, who was entering to visit the same patient. He gently pulled her aside and, with a touch of boldness, asked if she was married or in a serious relationship. She was bowled over by his charm and her blushing gave it all away. He asked if he could see her the next weekend, perhaps for a few drinks and dinner. She said she would be happy to. So that's how it began—and it soon turned into one of the wildest courtships in all of Statesboro. It was exciting. It was fun. And it was passionate.

Right from the start, they were madly and crazily in love. John wanted Dot's complete attention and total devotion, and she wanted to give it to him. Here were two people who grew up feeling for some reason that they were never really loved and now they felt it—they felt it right to the very core of their beings.

At the same time, they found they enjoyed drinking together, sometimes too much. Dot was often hung over after a date with John, but she was better at hiding how much she drank than he was—that is, except for one very embarrassing morning early in their courtship. The young nurse was awakened on the front lawn of the doctor's house on Lee Street by a dog licking her face and the milkman grinning down at her. John was lying nearby, sound asleep. She shook him and he slowly awakened with a big grin on his face. He looked around, recognized Dot's embarrassment, then grabbed her and pulled her close, saying, "Don't worry so much, darling. Everything's all right. Just pretend we're having an early morning picnic in the front yard."

It was part of the doctor's charm that he never seemed to worry about anything. He just took life as it came. Maybe it was the result of his war experiences, simply living life from one day to the next. But while Dot adored his charm and everything else about this talented and sometimes mysterious man, she was concerned about the direction in which their relationship was headed. Very, very concerned.

CHAPTER FIVE

A Loving Dilemma

DOROTHY CAROLYN RIGGS WOKE UP ONE MORNING AND DE-cided she couldn't marry Dr. Alfonso John Mooney. She made this momentous decision before even getting out of bed and actually tried as hard as she could to keep it once she was completely awake.

Indeed, she loved this man with all her heart and soul, more than she could put into words. But deep down, she felt like she didn't measure up to his standards—and particularly to the status of his well-known and highly respected family in the Statesboro community. She felt his family looked down on her, especially John's mother. That's why the young nurse would get so upset when he teased her every now and then while out drinking with friends. He'd wink and say, "I met Dot walking down a dirt road."

She was a simple country girl. He was an admired surgeon, a war hero, a man who had been married to a wealthy debutante who seemed to be everything she was not. If Sally Christian Spaulding wasn't enough to please him, what did a farmer's daughter from Jimps, Georgia, have to offer?

So as deeply and as passionately as she loved this man of her dreams, someone who swept her off her feet every chance he had, a handsome physician who proposed to her almost every time they embraced, she was determined not to marry him. And it wasn't just her own insecurities that plagued her or the warnings she was given by her mother and friends like Honey Bowen. She feared being drawn into a permanent relationship she wouldn't be able to handle, one that posed more questions than answers, an emotional firestorm that could possibly render her—a strong, self-determined young woman—totally powerless.

But she couldn't stop seeing him. And each time she did, her love for this charming and fascinating man only grew more intense.

In the midst of all her confusion, she decided to share her fears and concerns with Honey Bowen. She needed a friend she could confide in, someone older, wiser, and more mature—someone who knew both her and John quite well. Before Honey had her front door halfway open, Dot burst in and blurted out, "I love John so much but I think we're bad for each other. I don't know what to do about it. He keeps asking me to marry him. The next time he does, I don't think I can say no."

"Well, I think you had better say no, young lady," Honey quickly replied. "Love the man to death but for heaven's sake, don't marry him."

Honey had known John most of her life and she cared for him a great deal. But, being a close neighbor, she had also witnessed the changes in him ever since he returned home from the battlefield—how his drinking had increased, the obvious problems that led to his divorce, his comings and goings at all hours of the day and night. She was quite frank with her young friend, telling her she didn't think either one of them was ready to settle down and get married.

Dot remembered Honey Bowen's advice when she was sharing her experiences one day with some old friends later on in her life: "I always felt that marriage was sacred, that it was a commitment you made for life and you never broke commitments. I knew I needed to be careful about getting married because I didn't want to make a mistake. I have always been funny about making mistakes. I never wanted to make one.

"If I made a mistake, I wasn't about to admit it. And I knew it would be that way if I made the wrong decision about marriage. I would probably stay in it rather than admit I'd made a mistake."

But the real problem remained. Dot was honestly and truly in love. It wasn't a fantasy or some kind of hero worship. By now she had come to know John as a serious physician who loved his work and cared deeply for his patients. She saw the tender side of him that touched her heart, as well as the baffling and confusing side that concerned her. But in spite of all the partying, the drinking, the fun times, the dancing until dawn, she felt that love every time John looked at her, touched her, kissed her. And she knew he felt exactly the same way about her.

The other problem was that their love and their passion, combined with their drinking and their drugging—while not too serious as yet—still blinded them to what might lie ahead. They were unable to see that their love for each other and their love for their addictions were soon to collide—and how that powerful collision would create havoc in their lives.

It was around the first week of September 1947 when it all came to a head. They left the hospital early one afternoon and were driving to Savannah to have dinner at one of their favorite places, Johnny Harris's Supper Club. Just a few miles outside Statesboro, John suddenly pulled his car to the side of the road, turned off the engine, and grabbed Dot's hands. He looked intently into her eyes.

He told her again how much he worshipped her and the ground she walked on, but was frustrated that it always led to a dead-end street. He said he was also tired of proposing and that if she loved him half as much as he loved her, then she should make up her mind right there and then.

"I have a feeling that if we don't do it now, we'll never do it. Will you marry me, Dot?"

She fell into his arms, crying. "Yes, John. I'll marry you. I love you so much. So very, very much."

They drove the rest of the way to Savannah with Dot snuggled against her lover's arm. They had their favorite meal, rare T-bone steaks, celebrated with champagne, and danced until the supper club closed. The next day they took out a marriage license at City Hall and informed family and friends of their intentions to wed. They did, at the Bulloch County Courthouse on the afternoon of September 13, 1947.

Dot's father didn't go to the rather informal ceremony and small reception that followed. When Myrtis insisted they go, her husband simply slumped down into his front porch swing and grunted at his wife: "I reckon there ain't no point in me getting dressed up and going to town for that."

Arthur Riggs didn't fess up until some years later about the real reasons he refused to attend his daughter's marriage to John Mooney. First, John was a divorced man. Second, he drank too much too often. And third, he feared he'd get his little girl into a whole pack of trouble someday. The well-weathered farmer was right on all three counts.

So Myrtis went with her son and two other daughters, as did John's mother and his two sisters. Since the newlyweds could only take a few days off from work, they left the reception early and headed for a brief honeymoon on Tybee Island, Georgia, a well-known resort area just several hours away.

Its original inhabitants, the Euchee Indians, named the colorful and historic island eighteen miles southeast of Savannah "Tybee," which is the Euchee word for "salt."

In 1520, Spain laid claim to the island but didn't establish a colony there. So it soon became a den for pirates to hide from their pursuers and to use as a freshwater source. Then England invaded in the 1700s, Spain retreated, and Tybee Island became a peaceful and attractive British settlement—and later, after the American Revolution, one of Georgia's most popular recreation areas.

The island's strategic position near the mouth of the Savannah River made its northern tip an ideal location for a ninety-foot, brick and wood lighthouse. By the time John and Dot arrived to honeymoon there, the lighthouse had become one of the island's many popular tourist attractions.

On the southern tip was the Tybrisa Pavilion, a large dining and dancing hall that had also become a popular stop for big band tours. In between the northern tip and the southern tip were Fort Screven, the Revolutionary War historic district; the Tybee Post Theater, a home for summer stock; the Tybee Museum, which housed the island's historic archives; four first-class hotels; and a number of fine restaurants.

Tybee Island was not only an excellent choice for a honeymoon back in the 1940s, it was also a mecca for "snowbirds" during the harsh northern U.S. and Canadian winters. It had also become a much-sought-after vacation spot for people with asthma and allergies who thought the clean, saltwater breezes offered a special remedy for their ailments.

But it was September now. Most families had returned home to put their children back in school, and the "snowbirds" and allergy sufferers had not yet arrived. So it was very quiet and peaceful along the wide stretches of white sandy beaches and in the small resort town just beyond the rolling sand dunes. It gave the newlyweds from Statesboro time to pause, time to take a deep breath, to talk warmly, intimately, and sometimes even excitedly about the future. They would slow down, drink less, have a family, and live life the way most happily married couples did. That was their plan.

So what, as they danced through the night at the Tybee Pavilion, if they drank just a little too much? It was their honeymoon, an occasion to celebrate. It would be different once they returned home. They were both sure of that. In fact, they even toasted to their resolution during their last evening on Tybee Island.

It's often said that good intentions can be the best excuse for failure. And the now Mrs. Dorothy Riggs Mooney had the very best intentions one could possibly have when she and John arrived back in Statesboro to start their life together as husband and wife.

Even though the Lee Street house was almost twice the size of the farmhouse where she was born and raised, Dot knew she could take charge of the place and be a better homemaker than even her mother was, and without all the complaining. She soon discovered, however, that her new husband also liked to be in charge—that he enjoyed having things his own way. This was another one of those leftover traits from the war, when he found it necessary that his medical unit be run with only one commanding voice and no interference.

Everything ran smoothly until the day John ran out of liquor. That was the day he and his new bride reached their first accommodation. John decided he would handle all the finances and the liquor supplies, and Dot would handle the food shopping and the household chores. She quietly agreed. However, she quickly learned there wasn't much time for cleaning, shopping, and cooking together with her busy nursing schedule at the hospital. So the newlyweds sat down and reached their second accommodation. They hired some help. Through the recommendation of friends, Dot found a very pleasant and diligent churchgoing black lady named Martha who very quickly became an essential part of the family. And despite all the chaos that was soon to enter the Mooney household, Martha managed to handle it for the next seventeen years.

But for now, John and Dot's love was warm and alive and filled every moment they were together. Some nights Dot would lie in bed pressing her body against John's, watching him breathe. She would feel so very grateful that, despite all her partying before they met, she had clung to one of her most important principles.

She had never gotten so close to another man. She had drunk with men, partied with them, danced with them, but that was as far as it went. And she had certainly never done any of those things with other women's husbands.

At the same time, Dot felt she didn't need to know all the intimate details of her husband's past life: what it must have been like during the war . . . what it must have been like getting a divorce and all the questions and shame that come with it. She only needed to know that he loved her, and she knew in her heart that he did.

So deep down, despite her insecurities and concerns about the future, she was comforted by the fact that she could give herself and her love completely to this man lying beside her and not worry about anything he might find out about her. And maybe, just maybe, that would help them through any difficult personal times that might lie ahead.

Also, she respected John for trying to be a good member of the local Methodist church and attending services every Sunday despite being divorced and despite often being hungover after partying too much on Saturday night. The young physician still had a deep faith in God and at the same time wanted to keep up the outward pretenses of being a religious man. It was that constant struggle between what was true and what was put on that often caused him considerable guilt.

On the other hand, Dot still couldn't care less about church. She only went to be a good wife. The truth was, she continued to have the same terrible fear of God that she had had most of her life, and it only got worse at church services.

Looking back some years later, she believed her terrible fear came from being raised in what she called "a hard-shell, primitive fire-and-brimstone Baptist church" where the preacher insisted that everyone "fear the Lord." And she did, from that first day when her mother took her to church at the age of three weeks old right up to the present.

John Mooney had no such fear of God and no fear of church.

His only fear was that someone might smell the liquor on his breath as he sang loudly from his hymnal. He already sensed that the preacher had his own suspicions.

Since most of the residents of Statesboro continued to respect and admire the young surgeon, his medical practice grew. And he needed more help to handle the number of patients constantly crowding his office. Several times while he and Dot were court-ing, he had asked her to leave her job at the hospital and work for him. But she always refused. She loved the excitement at Bulloch County Hospital and the many different challenges she faced there each day. She also enjoyed the many friends she had made on the hospital staff. But now she was married to Dr. John Mooney, so when he asked her again shortly after they returned home from Tybee Island, she found it difficult to say no. In fact, she felt it was now her duty and responsibility to help her busy husband in any way she could.

So, since Martha was doing a fine job handling all the house-hold chores and putting a delicious dinner on the table every night, Dot was able to leave her job at the hospital—albeit with some reluctance—and help her doctor husband with his growing practice. She took over running the office, making appointments, giving shots, assisting with other patient needs, and sending out the bills. And before long, without her husband realizing it, she began discovering more about his "nonmedical activities" than she even at first suspected. And the more she learned, the more concerned she became—that is, until the day arrived when she found she could use some of those same "nonmedical activities" to solve her own problems and fulfill her own needs.

Even though she drank at home with her husband, Dot was unaware that his alcohol consumption had been gradually increas-ing again. She never counted his drinks. She was also unaware that the young physician had promised himself years ago that he would never be a "drunk doctor"—a physician treating patients while intoxicated. And he knew he was nearing that threshold. So he found a solution. It was a solution that didn't completely surprise his wife when she discovered it. But it was a solution both knew was terribly wrong—that is, unless you added a strong potion of denial and self-deception to the mix.

The solution? John switched from alcohol to selective drugs to get through the day. He no longer drank in the morning when operating or early afternoon when seeing patients. And in his mind, he was keeping his promise. He was not a "drunk doctor."

John started off slowly at first, taking small amounts of narcotics, tranquilizers, and sedatives, trying to find what he would come to call "the balanced life." Arriving home from the office, he would drink until bedtime, then take some tranquilizers to help him sleep. In the morning before leaving the house, he would take amphetamines to wake up. Then he'd take codeine for his hangover from the night before. But that made him sick. So he'd take Bromanyl and barbital to stop the nausea, but they made him sleepy and he'd take Benzedrine to keep awake. But Benzedrine made him jittery and nervous, so he took Nembutal to calm his nerves. His favorite was Doriden because that made everything all right with the world. Some years later when he was clean and sober, John would say with tongue in cheek, "I fell in love with Doriden. I called it my churchgoing medicine. Since I was afraid some parishioners might smell alcohol on my breath, I'd take four Doriden tablets before leaving for church instead of having a few drinks. By the time I got there I felt so comfortable it was like sitting six inches above your pew. Time would whiz by. The preacher's sermon only seemed to last three minutes and I was suddenly back outside with the crowd. I felt like I was walking with both feet planted firmly in midair.

"I soon discovered, though, that you can't take these medications for granted. They'll play tricks on you. When eating, you have to watch the fork all the way into your mouth so you don't stab yourself in the eye. And when you tie your shoes you have to be careful you don't tie the laces of one shoe together with the laces of the other shoe. You can trip and hurt yourself. And you

have to make sure the buttons of your shirt are in the right but-
tonholes. It's the sacrifices you have to make to lead this 'balanced
life.'"

While Dot would see her husband taking what he called "some
pick-me-ups" in the morning, she had no idea his intake of drugs
during the day was increasing. Or maybe she really didn't want to
see it. Besides, there were few outward signs in his work with patients or comments about it in the hospital operating room. Most
people who knew John knew he drank, but they also believed he
would never let it interfere with his practicing medicine. Quite
apropos of this point, there was a story circulating around town
about that time concerning an exchange between two of John's
patients:

"I saw Dr. Mooney leaving a restaurant yesterday and he seemed
a bit tipsy. It made me feel just a little concerned. What do you
think?"

The other patient replied: "I'd rather have a drunk Dr. Mooney
operate on me any day than any sober surgeon in town."

It was late one afternoon when John came out of his office and
took his wife aside. She was startled by his appearance. His face
was pale and sweating, and he seemed to have trouble catching
his breath. He said he had to go home right away and rest—that
she should tend to whatever patients she could and have the others come back another day. Then he walked unsteadily down the
hall and out of the building.

Caught off guard, Dot didn't know what to do at first. The
waiting room was crowded. Where should she begin? Should she
run after her husband to make sure he was all right, or should
she stay and care for the patients? She decided to tell everyone a
little white lie: that Dr. Mooney had to rush off to an emergency
and wouldn't be back for the rest of the day. She then apologized,
rescheduled their appointments, and finally called the house to
see how John was doing. Martha said he was resting on the living
room sofa and seemed to be perfectly fine.

The young nurse hung up the phone, took a deep breath, and then quickly rose from behind her desk. That's when she felt it, that nervous, tingling sensation in her arms, the weakness in her legs, that feeling of bewilderment and anxiety in her head. She quickly sat down, hoping it would pass. But it didn't.

As she tried to regain control of her emotions, Dot suddenly realized this was the same kind of panic attack she used to get as a young nursing student in Savannah. She used to call them her "nervous spells." It was one of the reasons she decided to leave nursing school and return home. The attack went away after a few minutes, but she sat there wondering why these feelings had suddenly returned now.

As a nurse at Bulloch County Hospital, she had cared for many people who suffered similar episodes. Few could explain or understand why. The doctors would prescribe tranquilizers and they seemed to calm things down quite well. So she thought, if it worked for them, why not give it a try? She didn't realize, perhaps, that she was about to "self-medicate," a dangerous procedure her husband was trying to perfect for himself.

Dot rose more carefully this time and made her way slowly to the prescription cabinet in her husband's office. She had a key. She opened the cabinet, took out a sample box of Miltown, and edged to the sink. She opened the box and swallowed two pills. She put another sample box in her jacket pocket, then closed and locked the cabinet. She stood there quietly for a few minutes and then began to breathe much easier. She turned out the lights, left the office, and went home thinking she had solved another problem in her life.

As for John, there were evenings when Dot was off visiting her family in Jimps or having dinner with girlfriends. He would sit in a chair on the back porch at Lee Street all by himself, drinking. He was now putting away more than a fifth of liquor each night. Every now and then he would be overwhelmed by a sense of anxiety, a fear that all he had studied for, all that he had worked so hard and so diligently to achieve, was slowly slipping away. Then an alcoholic stupor would engulf him and a melancholy mood would set in. The onetime war hero would see himself enjoying one of those rare respites of calm and quiet on the battlefront, stepping outside his field hospital tent for a quick smoke. He'd stand there thinking about what it was going to be like when he finally got home. He would swear that all he wanted was a small taste of the good things in life—to be a good doctor, a good husband, a good father, a good citizen, a good churchgoing man. If that could happen, he'd be so grateful he'd never ask God for another thing. Then the artillery would start up again and the B-17 bombers would roar overhead. He'd grind his cigarette out in the dirt, duck back into the tent, and continue performing lifesaving surgery on his wounded and bloody soldiers.

Sometimes his eyes would moisten as he came out of the stupor, realizing he had been back in Statesboro for quite some time now and that all those things he desired he either already had or they were within his reach. That's when he knew where the fear was coming from. Yes, he wanted those good things in life all right, but he wanted to drink whiskey and take drugs too. He sensed it might be the whiskey and the drugs that were slowly pulling those good things from his grasp. In his heart he knew he couldn't have all the good things in life and drink and drug at the same time. And when he rose from his porch chair and headed upstairs to his bedroom, he was always afraid to ask himself the most important question of all: what was it he wanted more?

At the same time, John was convinced he wasn't an alcoholic. He had asked himself that question many times and always came up with the same answer. He knew alcoholics. He had seen them many times. He had treated some. They were men in threadbare overcoats who wore scraggly beards and slept in doorways. He was a respected doctor who lived in a lovely home with a lovely wife and successfully treated many patients. He was far from being a bum or a hobo like they were.

As a matter of fact, from the outside looking in, everything seemed rather normal on Lee Street and very compatible between the young physician and his new wife. Things were good, he thought. Things certainly weren't the same as they once were. There was a time when John used to blame his drinking on his first wife, Sally, a woman who never seemed satisfied with anything— his medical practice, where they lived, their circle of friends. So he found a few drinks relieved the pressure. Drinking relieved his unhappiness. It gave him an escape from his misery and frustration. At least that's what he told himself.

With Dot it was different. She was a loving, warm, and comforting drinking companion who understood her husband's needs and tried her best to satisfy them. And that's how she felt too— that drinking with her husband strengthened the bond between them, expanded their mutual understanding, and, for a time at least, heated their passion.

On Valentine's Day of 1948 Dot announced to John that she was pregnant with their first child. He was ecstatic. She was surprised. She thought for a while that they would not be able to have children. After all, John had been married for ten years to Sally and they had no children. So she was relieved that they could have a family—but she was also very concerned.

Although all of the scientific details of what is today called fetal alcohol syndrome were not known in the late 1940s, Dot was well aware that drinking alcohol and taking drugs could have deleterious effects on a developing fetus. Actually, the young nurse had seen for herself some of those effects when assisting in deliveries at the hospital—retarded growth, poor lung development, vision problems, shaking and tremors, and serious heart defects that sometimes led to the infant's death.

So Dot stopped drinking and taking drugs immediately and spent the next seven months fearing the worst while hoping for the best.

CHAPTER SIX

Another New Start

"I ALWAYS THOUGHT IT WAS QUITE UNBECOMING FOR A MAN OF some stature in the community to be tipsy in public, and even more so in front of his wife's family, especially when she's carrying his baby. As his sister-in-law, I thought it was simply a disgrace."

While Marilyn Riggs is today one of the late John Mooney's biggest admirers, she had little respect for him when he first married into the Riggs family. "Almost every time I saw him, he was always acting silly and stupid, probably because he was drinking," she added. "Some people thought he was funny. I didn't."

Marilyn, another country girl from Jimps, Georgia, married Dot's older brother, Arthur James, who was fifteen years older than Marilyn. She would often josh: "I was probably the only person my husband could have married that could get along with his mother, Myrtis. Despite her being a domineering woman, I just never let her bother me. But for some reason, with Dr. John, it was different."

While Dot drove out to Jimps quite often to visit her family, John would go along with her only on holidays or special occasions like birthdays and weddings. But even though Marilyn didn't see him that often, Dot's husband seemed to raise her hackles every time he showed up at the Riggses' farmhouse.

"God forgive me for saying it, but I always felt like he sort of grew up thinking he was someone special, that he seemed to have a way of looking down at folks he didn't particularly relate to," she said, trying to explain her feelings back then. "Maybe that's because back in those days, people thought doctors were some kind of gods. I know a lot of his patients thought that way about him."

Marilyn's remarks were closer to the mark than even she knew. John himself admitted later in life that he really enjoyed playing God as a doctor—that at times in his drunken arrogance and egotism he would actually believe he held the power of life and death over his patients. He said it became one of those profound character defects he had to work hard at getting rid of in order to stay sober. He also had to stop playing God with everyone around him, including himself.

As he once said, "I also thought I was different from other people—that I didn't have the same reaction to pills and drugs as they did.

"I would prescribe medications for patients, telling them to be sure to follow the directions, like take one capsule every six hours by the clock. Then I'd take a handful of the same thing and not be concerned about the reaction. I'd brush it off, or take another medication to counteract the reaction of the first one.

"It's lunatic to think you're different, but that's what I believed about myself—that I was a doctor and I knew more than anyone else. Part of it was my ego and the other part was the liquor and drugs. And maybe there was a third part—the fact that I didn't get killed during the war made me feel like I was Superman. Who knows?"

There was something else that also affected the physician's attitude, something he had difficulty admitting even to himself. He expected life to be easier once he came home from the war and it wasn't. Sure, there was no longer any shooting and bombing or mud ruts and freezing cold, but the pressure on him seemed to be mounting just the same.

By the time he arrived back in Statesboro, John knew the practice of medicine had become quite a lucrative field for most doctors, and especially for good surgeons like him. And by now he was an excellent and very experienced surgeon. He felt that once you work hard to get your medical degree, all you needed then was to get a stethoscope, a ballpoint pen, and a prescription pad and you could make an excellent living anywhere—and live a life of relative ease. That is, unless you drank and drugged too much. That could complicate things.

Indeed, John was making very good money, but he wasn't saving any. He handled money like there was no tomorrow. Between his drinking, drugging, and his love for fancy new cars and other "toys," he was starting to pile up some debt. And since he was the one handling the finances, Dot was unaware of any potential problems.

But now they were expecting their first child. The young physician knew things couldn't go on like this. If ever there were a time and a reason to change the direction of his life, to make another new start and be the kind of husband and father he knew he should be, it was now. Yes, it would take another determined effort. He would have to use every ounce of willpower and self-control he could muster just as he did when his ex-wife left him. But he could do it. He knew he could.

Then, as quickly as he made his decision to stop altogether, John amended that decision to "slowing down." His problem was not his drinking and drugging, he told himself, but drinking and drugging too much. For example, he didn't need almost two fifths of liquor every day. A few glasses of wine at dinnertime should be more than sufficient. And by "slowing down," he could also eliminate some of the drugs from his "balanced life" routine. Yes, that was it. He would control his intake and everything would be fine.

For Dot, it was different. She wasn't drinking or drugging at all, and that only made her already difficult pregnancy worse. Now in her seventh month, she was always uncomfortable. She felt she was putting on too much weight, her feet were swelling, and she was frequently fighting off panic attacks. She would sit and read books or play her favorite records. But neither of these activities relieved her "nervous spells," which John called her "bitchy moods." She felt sorry for herself and only John's loving arms could calm her and make her feel a little better.

One afternoon, her blood pressure suddenly shot sky high. She got dizzy and almost passed out. Concerned about both Dot and the baby, Martha quickly called an ambulance. At the hospital Dot was rushed into the delivery room and, because of her high blood pressure and heart palpitations, labor was induced. She delivered her first son prematurely. They named him Alfonso after his grandfather, but everyone simply called him Al.

Dot was relieved to know that her baby, though almost two months premature, was born healthy. However, because he was so underweight, he had to remain in the hospital for more than a month before he could come home. His young mother felt sad and a bit guilty, but once she tucked him into the brand-new crib in his beautifully decorated nursery room at Lee Street, she didn't hesitate at all to resume her drinking routine.

At the same time, the joy of having his first child, and particularly a son, helped John in his latest attempt to control his own drug and liquor intake—at least for a while. He enjoyed coming home from his office to play with his son, to hold him, and at times to even change his diaper. All the while he'd tease his wife about being an "idler," telling her how much all the patients missed her tender treatment and that her replacement—a practical nurse named Ruby Blizzard—wasn't nearly as efficient. He said perhaps he needed another nurse to better handle the job and keep the patients happy like Dot used to do. Then he would put their son back into his crib, hug his wife, and head for the dining room for another one of Martha's delicious meals.

Each night they would finish a bottle of wine with their dinner and another before going to bed. For a while, John felt very satisfied with himself and his self-control as he snuggled under the covers to make love to this woman he so adored. Little did he know that his wife felt quite differently. She was totally unsatisfied with her own inability to cut back, to control her own intake. And, while she enjoyed making mad passionate love with her husband, she was deeply fearful of getting pregnant again because of her drinking. This was something she was reluctant to share with him, particularly when he held her so close in his arms.

Dot did her best to be a good mother but was very grateful to have Martha there to help, not only with the household chores but with the baby as well. Some mornings, after she secretly had had too much the night before, she would sleep really late. Other mornings she would be up early to prepare little Al for another trip to Jimps. Dot loved showing the baby off to her mother and father as well as to the rest of the family. And the fact that she could hold off drinking or taking any drugs until she returned home late in the afternoon convinced her she wasn't nearly as addicted as she sometimes thought she might be.

But then there was an incident that really made her stop and think. She had asked her husband's sister Sarah and Sarah's husband, Bert, to watch the baby while Dot and John went to a party with some friends. Her sister-in-law loved little Al, so she and Bert eagerly accepted the invitation. The Mooneys got ready for the party the usual way—by having one too many drinks before they left.

When Sarah arrived at the house with her husband, the baby was crying. Dot said he probably had gas from drinking his bottle too quickly and just needed to be rocked to sleep. Then she left. The young child began crying even louder despite being in Sarah's tender arms. Bert got particularly upset and asked his wife to check the baby's diaper. Sarah was shocked to discover that Dot had put one of the safety pins right through the infant's skin.

The relatives were fully prepared to chastise their sister-in-law.

By the time she and John arrived home from the party, they were both so inebriated that her in-laws realized any rebuke at the time would have fallen on deaf ears. So Sarah waited until the next day, when she spoke on the phone to a very contrite mother who swore something like that had never happened before and would never happen again.

But there was another incident that made Dot Mooney wonder even more about a possible addiction. It was an embarrassing event the young mother would not forget for a long time and one her brother's wife, Marilyn, would never forget.

"I think it happened on one of those summer holidays, possibly the Fourth of July," Marilyn recalled. "Anyway, we were having a family picnic down at the pond not far from the farmhouse where my husband and I lived. It was right next door to the Riggses. I remember Dr. John came along that day with Dot and the baby. I think little Al was about a year old at the time."

She said there was plenty of beer and moonshine at the picnic together with barbecue and watermelon. But no one got drunk except for John and Dot. They were waving American flags, laughing out loud, and "acting rather rowdy." Then they decided to take a boat ride on the pond.

"Both of them got into this little old pond boat and Dr. John started to paddle away from the shore," Marilyn explained. "Dot had the baby in her arms. They were acting real silly and happy-go-lucky. A lot of folks were laughing too, but not my husband, Jim. He seemed really concerned.

"As I watched, I saw them rocking back and forth in the boat. Suddenly it turned over and they all fell into the pond. Fortunately the water was only waist deep. I saw Dr. John take the baby from Dot as she started splashing around. That's when my husband, her brother, jumped into the pond, grabbed Dot by the arm, and pulled her to shore.

"Then they started arguing. Soaking wet but arguing. Dot could get real nasty back then if she didn't agree with you. I guess she thought it was all a big joke, but her brother didn't."

But John also thought it was real funny. He was roaring with laughter as he waded ashore with his son in his arms. Still, the incident put a damper on the picnic. People started to pack up and leave.

"Strangely enough, there really wasn't much danger involved," Marilyn concluded, "since the pond was so shallow. Except you knew they were drinking and anything could have happened. I used to wonder why people did those foolish kinds of things. I still do."

Dot remained unconcerned about the whole incident until a few weeks later, when she learned she was pregnant again. It wasn't bad enough that she was still drinking and taking drugs, but she now realized her lack of willpower and worried that her foolish actions at the pond could have harmed her unborn baby.

Once again John comforted her. He told her that as a doctor, he was sure everything would be all right. His confidence was reassuring and his delight over having another child made her very happy indeed—that is, until she thought about the struggle she was facing to stop her liquor and pills one more time and prove again she didn't have an addiction.

Dot's other struggle was trying to hide her actual intake from her husband. She felt she was being quite successful and that John thought she only drank when they were together and had no idea about the drugs she was taking. That's why she felt somewhat hypocritical when she would speak to him about his drinking, since he never expressed any concern about hers—even after the boat incident at the family picnic.

But Dot was really beginning to worry about her husband. Whenever she raised the subject, he would agree that he had to slow down again, not just because they were having another baby, but also because it was now affecting his medical practice. His nurse, Ruby Blizzard, was also threatening to leave and he had to start looking for a replacement.

Added to these growing problems, he was now getting to the

hospital late for surgery some mornings and causing a snag in the operating room schedule. The other surgeons hadn't complained as yet, but he knew it was only a matter of time.

Dot suggested that maybe her husband was much too focused on his practice and his family and that it might be making him too tense. Perhaps he needed other things in his life to relax him, like some hobbies, for example. John thought that was a great idea, and before the week was out, he was deeply involved in photography.

"When I did something, I usually went all out," John Mooney would often brag. "I would become almost obsessed with whatever it was. That's what happened with my photography too.

"First I built me a professional, fully equipped dark room in an upstairs room of the house. Then I went out and bought about a dozen cameras and a ton of film. I began shooting pictures all over the place, the house, the yard, mostly of Dot and the baby and also when we would occasionally take a ride somewhere. I was very pleased at how fast I developed some expertise with a camera.

"But the dark room was my downfall. I would sit in there and drink a fifth of Scotch for every pint of developing solution I used. I either underdeveloped or overdeveloped most of the pictures I took. I ruined more film than I care to talk about before I finally gave up that hobby."

Their second son, Jimmy Mooney, was born on April 24, 1950. He was born with a rare intestinal problem and needed major surgery. Dr. Bird Daniel, a good friend of John's and an excellent general surgeon, waited six weeks in order to give the newborn child a chance to recover from a difficult delivery. Then he operated and the surgery had a very successful outcome.

Almost losing their second son made a fearful and painful impression on both parents. They were now determined to quit drinking and drugging for good. They finally recognized it could destroy their family as well as all their hopes and dreams. But what they didn't realize was that by now, they were both suffering from an insidious and incurable disease—an addiction to alcohol and drugs. While they thought they could stop or at least control it, they had no idea they were now powerless to do so.

Despite botching his venture into photography, John decided to give this hobby thing one more chance. He had always enjoyed reading *Popular Mechanics,* so he thought he might like building things. He chose woodworking as his next attempt to spice up his life. He thought it would occupy his mind and hopefully sop up the time at home when he would usually be drinking. It seemed like a good plan.

Going all out once again, the determined physician bought several thousand dollars' worth of Delta power tools—band saws, grinders, drill presses, lathes, and all kinds of hand tools. He put them all in his garage, which he turned into a workshop. Then he actually began to build things like an armchair and a small dresser. However, it wasn't long before the initial fervor wore off and he was taking a bottle of Scotch along with him to stimulate his woodworking chores.

Sometimes John would be in his noisy workshop until midnight, sipping on his bottle and running a few small pieces of lumber through his band saw because he liked the kind of gentle hum it made. At other times he'd turn on all thirteen of his machines and sip himself into a trance until the neighbors called and complained. Then Dot would march down to the workshop and get him. They often argued furiously all the way into the house and sometimes for hours afterward.

John disliked arguing and confrontation, but Dot grew up with it. And now things were getting on her nerves and she didn't know what else to do. She knew her husband was starting to lie to her about certain things, and the one thing she hated was lying. How can you trust anyone when they lie to you? she thought. So she would yell at him when he made up stories about the lack of money or where he went some days after he left the office or really how much he was drinking and taking drugs. Still, she could only yell or argue for so long before the sense of her own hypocrisy would return.

It was less than a month after little Jimmy was born that John finally found a replacement for Ruby Blizzard. Her name was Dallas Cason. She was a unique and experienced nurse, who not only would serve this very troubled physician faithfully and professionally for many years, but in the end would help save his medical practice and his life as well.

A native of Claxton, Georgia, and a graduate of the Georgia Baptist Hospital's nursing school in Atlanta, Dallas married an army officer who kept moving from one military base to another. As a result, she had great nursing skills developed at excellent hospitals in Alabama, Arizona, California, and Georgia. After her husband left the service, they came back to Georgia and settled down in Claxton, which is about twenty-five miles from Statesboro.

Shortly after the Casons moved into their new home, Dallas's neighbor dropped by to welcome her. By sheer coincidence, she just happened to work for Dr. Bird Daniel, John's good friend who operated on his son, Jimmy.

"When I told her that I was also a nurse and was looking for a position," Dallas explained, "my neighbor said she might be able to help. She said she knew a Doctor John Mooney in Statesboro who needed an office nurse but wondered if I'd be willing to travel that far. I asked her if she could tell me more about this Dr. Mooney."

The neighbor seemed to hesitate for a moment, then replied, "Well, he is very intelligent. He's a kind and good man and he's a very good surgeon. But he has one problem. He drinks."

Dallas smiled. "If he's a good man and a good doctor, the driving distance and his imbibing won't bother me. I'll go to work in the morning and I'll come home at night and what he does with his time won't have anything to do with me."

Little did she know what lay ahead.

Dallas Cason went to work for Dr. Mooney on May 15, 1950. She was challenged right from the outset. Only on the job a few months, she found herself one day with a waiting room filled with patients and no Dr. Mooney. The experienced nurse was not someone given to panic. She had already gotten to know Dot quite well and loved her from the start. So, trying to decide what to do, Dallas called the doctor's wife to ask where her husband might be. To her surprise, Dot was brutally frank and honest.

"Your guess is as good as mine. He may show up soon or he may not show up at all. I suggest you wait a short time and if he doesn't make an appearance, tell the patients that Dr. John forgot to mention he had to leave this morning for a doctor's convention. I'll make sure that little white lie is on my soul, not yours."

The fact is, John had gone off on a real bad bender this time. He had come out of a blackout in a small hotel in Binghamton, New York. There was an airline ticket on the bed, but he had no recollection of flying there. He decided to take a bus home but came out of another blackout in another motel, this one in Macon, Georgia.

Fearing he might never get home, and not knowing what to tell his wife, his new office nurse, or his patients, the hungover physician called his preacher in Statesboro. He confessed that he had messed things up and begged for the preacher's help and direction.

The preacher told John to stay where he was, that he would drive over and bring him home. He said he would also call his wife and tell her he was all right. Fortunately the distressed surgeon had half a bottle of liquor left, so he was able to calm his nerves and take a shower while waiting for the compassionate clergyman to arrive.

On the way back to Statesboro, the preacher thought he was speaking to a humbled and contrite man who had learned his lesson. But he wasn't.

"John," he said quite frankly, "your problem is you think you're something special . . . that you can do things like this and get away with it. You think you don't react like other people and that you have certain talents and characteristics that other people don't have. What you have to realize is that you're nobody but plain old John Mooney. That's all you are. You're just like everybody else."

He was shocked by his companion's reply: "Preacher, I'd like to believe you, but it's just not true."

While John displayed his arrogance and ego in the preacher's car, he was a very humble man walking into the front door of his Lee Street home, where he was greeted by a wife who was frustrated and bewildered one more time. But soon they patched things up and it was going to be another one of those new beginnings. The result—Dot got pregnant again, only this time she had a miscarriage two months later. It weighed heavily on her mind since she was convinced it was caused by her drinking and drugging. Her husband tried to convince her otherwise but she could tell he wasn't all that sure himself.

Dr. John Mooney was unaware that he was on an elevator with buttons, thinking he could push one and get off at any floor he chose. He had no idea how close he was getting to the basement. Despite clinging to his arrogance and threads of ego, he did sense his troubles were only getting worse. That's when he began to make the rounds of psychiatrists and psychiatric hospitals. He went from Atlanta to New York, from Kentucky to Florida, trying desperately to find someone who could explain what was wrong with his mind, what was it that caused him to drink so much and take drugs even when he didn't want to take them. What was driving him to the edge of insanity?

No one could convince the skilled surgeon that he was an alcoholic and a drug addict. He was certain there was something wrong with his brain. Maybe he injured it during the war. Perhaps he was born with a brain wired the wrong way so that he couldn't control his desire to get high, to do things that hurt himself and all those around him.

John kept searching and searching, but he just couldn't find that one doctor who might have the answer for him.

"I never found that doctor," John once said. "I don't think any addict ever will. There is no such animal. If this thing could be resolved through psychiatry, then I wouldn't have to drink so much or take so much dope. Besides, I don't think I was ever really looking for a life of complete abstinence then, or thought it was even possible for me to live without a drink. Maybe I felt that life would be too boring or too painful."

He once told a close friend exactly how he felt at that particular time in his life: "I was like a man who saw a boat lying on a riverbank. As I climbed in, the boat began to drift away from the shore. Suddenly I realized the boat had no paddles or anchor. So I just sat there not knowing what to do. I realized that if the boat wasn't stopped by some obstruction in the river, it could drift all the way out into the ocean and soon I'd be lost. Yet I just sat there."

The only anchor John believed he had left at this point was Dot . . . her love . . . her caring . . . her belief that somehow, in some way, things would work out. He needed her now more than ever and she needed him. So they opened their arms to each other. They loved each other desperately—even though they loved their addictions too. And, as had been the case since the day they met, neither of them could see how these two loves were on a collision course in their lives or envision the chaos they were bound to bring.

On May 6, 1953, Dot gave birth to their third son, Robert Mooney. She had been praying as best she knew how, and her prayers were answered. Little Bobby was born the healthiest of their three sons. But he was born into a household that was getting more dysfunctional by the day.

As far as his medical practice was concerned, John loved to brag to his fellow physicians that he had found the best nurse in the state of Georgia to handle his office and his patients. But while he touted Dallas Cason's experience and abilities, he stopped short of telling anyone how well she was taking care of him.

And she was, even though his new nurse had two-year-old twin daughters at home. She was able to give her boss all the time he needed to maintain his medical practice because she had a kind and generous mother-in-law to watch after them.

"My mother-in-law loved my girls," Dallas explained. "Also, she lived nearby so I would drop them off at her house every morning on my way to work and pick them up on my way home. If I was running a bit late in the evening, either she or my husband would feed them and get them ready for bed. So I had no worries driving to and from work—only when I got to the office."

Dallas never knew what to expect. If the doctor was at the hospital in the morning performing scheduled surgery, she would open the mail, check the day's appointments, and generally get things ready for his patient load in the afternoon. If he had no surgery scheduled and was not in the office when she arrived or shortly after, she would wait until the morning patients grew antsy, then she would call Dot. If neither of them had any idea where he might be, then Dallas would conjure up a plan to cope with the situation.

After a while, the inventive nurse had the good Dr. Mooney having so many cases of hay fever or the flu or attending so many doctor conventions or medical education programs that his patients came to believe he was either the most allergic doctor in town or the smartest physician in Georgia.

One evening at Lee Street after Martha had gone and Dot was putting the children to bed, she heard a loud crash from downstairs. It sounded as if someone had fallen. Then she heard a series of painful grunts and groans and knew immediately that something had happened to her husband. She quickly put six-month-old Bobby in his crib and rushed down the steps to find John rolling around on the living room floor. He had apparently fallen off a chair and was foaming at the mouth.

Having treated many seizures and convulsions at the hospital, the experienced nurse knew exactly what to do. She had all the necessary medications in the house. Within minutes, the physician began to regain his senses. But Dot sat on the floor with his head in her lap for sometime, wiping his face with a wet towel. Her own face was deathly pale and tears ran down her cheeks. John began to breathe easier. Suddenly little Bobby started to cry rather loudly. She helped her husband to the sofa, eased him back onto a pillow, and laid the moistened towel across his forehead. Then she went to tend her son.

Her husband was more coherent when Dot returned, which eased her fears quite a bit. She sat on the sofa, once again resting his head on her lap. He said he didn't want to go to the hospital because he knew what caused the convulsion and that maybe he had finally had the wake-up call he needed. As she ran her fingers through his hair, John said he had to go somewhere to get really "cleaned out"—some treatment center where he might possibly find a way to lick his problem or at least better control it.

Yes, Dot thought, her husband had said the same things to her before, but he had never sounded this serious. And he had never seemed this frightened before. As much as she didn't want to raise her hopes, she couldn't help feeling the butterflies fluttering inside.

In John's prior search for his sanity, the now-beaten surgeon had heard about a psychiatric facility in New Canaan, Connecticut, called Silver Hill, a swanky place but one said to have a good record of success working with professional people. So, despite the fact that he really couldn't afford it, off he went.

The large white building was settled into green rolling hills dotted with tall oaks and spreading elms. And the flowers and shrubs that lined the long cement drive gave the treatment center a welcoming, peaceful feeling. Perhaps that's why the still red-eyed physician had a sense of ease and good expectations as he stepped from the courtesy van that had picked him up at the airport.

Several smiling staff members greeted him and led him into a thickly carpeted admitting room. It was certainly the kind of welcome a highly respected surgeon from Georgia deserved. At least that was John's first fleeting thought, which lasted until he was accompanied down the tiled hallway and started to notice some of his gaunt, yellowish, red-faced, unsmiling fellow patients.

One of the staff members who had greeted him led the physician to his large, comfortable room. After showing the new patient the dresser and closet for his clothes and the elegant bathroom with fluffy white towels, soap, and shampoo, the staff member handed John a big, thick book with a red-and-yellow dust jacket; the book was titled *Alcoholics Anonymous.*

"Read it," the middle-aged man suggested in a kind voice. "You might even like it."

As the newly arrived physician explained, "I did read it, and I did like it. I remember thinking, this is a wonderful book for alcoholics, and I know many alcoholics back in Statesboro. I'm going to bring some copies of this book home and give it to them.

"But I saw nothing in that book for me. There are stories in that thing that are right down the line like mine, but I did not see it."

And that's how it started off at the swanky psychiatric hospital in New Canaan, Connecticut.

During the sixty days or so that John remained at the facility, he underwent intensive psychotherapy. He was told he was completely disorganized, that he had to get some order back into his life. Any doctor who makes his hospital rounds at three o'clock in the morning and wakes his patients up to ask them how they feel, he was told, sounds like he's just a bit off kilter.

And when John's life in general was put under a microscope, he was amazed at how out of bounds it really was. He would come home from making his rounds about 5:00 a.m., have too many drinks, and go to bed. He'd wake very late so that his morning office hours would be pushed back into the afternoon, upsetting many of his patients.

Sometimes he'd have a light lunch followed by some pills. He would then confer with his office nurse about the next day's schedule, assuring her he would be on time for all his appointments. Then he would go home, get drunk, often not have any dinner, and start the next day the very same way.

"You have to get yourself onto a regular schedule," his counselor insisted. "You have to get up early in the morning, do a bit of exercising, eat breakfast, avoid even the smallest drink or pill, and get to your appointments on time. If you lead a normal, organized life, help others, and contribute to society, then your self-esteem will grow and you will have no need to drink or drug to make yourself feel better."

It all made perfect sense. By the time the physician was ready to leave Silver Hill, he had been clean and sober for more than two months, was in much better physical health, and was filled with a great deal of self-confidence. And he was eager and excited to get back home to start better organizing his life.

Dot's growing hope turned into a glowing faith when she saw the look on her husband's face and listened intently to the positive things he was saying. Her faith grew even more when he climbed out of bed at seven the next morning and went for a jog. She just knew this was an important turning point in their lives.

John not only planned and followed an organized routine at home, but made sure it carried over into his professional life. He was at the hospital early for his surgical appointments and back in his office in plenty of time to care for his waiting patients. Dallas was more than pleased to see how he had changed and quite relieved that she no longer had to add to her list of white lies to protect her boss.

On Saturday mornings the physician would play golf with some of his fellow doctors and later take his family for a ride in his white Thunderbird convertible. On Sundays he was now teaching

Bible studies at his church. But most important he was staying off liquor, pills, and narcotics. He once told a good friend, "I'm a guy who can get hooked on anything. For a while there, I thought I was finally getting hooked on the good things in life."

But the now-sober surgeon still had a few things twisting and turning in his gut. He resented that all of his patients hadn't come back to him. He blamed it on some of the other doctors in town. He felt they were talking about him and the things he used to do. Also, at times he would pass people on the streets of Statesboro and if they didn't respond to his warm smile and pleasant hello, he would think they held something against him. John would feel a twinge of anger.

A year had gone by and he still hadn't had a drink of liquor or taken any drugs. He felt good about himself. And at home, Dot had also cut down significantly on her own consumption. The children were healthy and getting bigger by the day. So, despite his occasional bouts with self-pity and resentment, all seemed to be right with the world.

John had just returned from playing golf one day when he accidentally slammed the car door shut on his left index finger. The pain was excruciating. Convinced he had broken the finger, he drove over to his office and took an X-ray. Sure enough the finger was severely fractured. He wrapped it in a splint and headed home.

That night the pain grew even worse. He told his wife that if he didn't take something for the pain, he wouldn't be able to sleep. So she went into the bathroom, took some Demerol from a small cabinet, and gave it to him. Since he had been clean and sober for over a year now, she thought nothing of it.

Some years later John was able to joke about what happened as a result of that night and his injured finger, but that was only after the past no longer controlled their lives. He would say with a slight smile, "I thought I had read somewhere that when a narcotics addict is rehabilitated, it is safe for him to take narcotics in the case of a severe emergency but only if it is administered under the direction of a physician. Well, I thought, I'm a physician. So I will take a hundred milligrams of Demerol very carefully for my pain, which I did. Then I took another hundred milligrams of Demerol the next morning just in case the pain might come back."

And that's how the wheels of addiction started rolling again and that's how Dr. John Mooney's organized life fell to pieces one more time. He was still unaware that he was heading down on that elevator and was getting closer and closer to the basement.

CHAPTER SEVEN

Even Chaos Can Seem Normal

ALTHOUGH SHE WAS SHATTERED EMOTIONALLY ONCE AGAIN BY her husband's slip back into his addictions after such a long period of sobriety, Dot Mooney handled the situation the way most addicted people do. She increased her own consumption. She felt it helped her drown her sorrows and ward off encroaching fears of the future.

Even though things seemed to be falling down around her, she was still determined to be the best mother she could be to their three sons while at the same time trying to hide her habit from them and the rest of the outside world. She and John made a pact that they would never drink in front of the children. However, they rarely considered what effect their erratic behavior was having when they would get intoxicated practically every evening and sometimes wind up in drunken arguments. Often Dot would wake up in the morning not remembering what happened the night before. Other times she would be so hungover the children would have to wake her to get their breakfast. That's why she began having Martha come to the house earlier every morning.

As Al, Jimmy, and Bobby grew older their mother took them to Sunday school, "because that was the right thing for a mother to do." While the class was in progress, she would sit in a corner of the church nursery with her head down and her hand covering her mouth in order to block out the stench of the liquor on her breath. Nevertheless, life was slowly becoming a confusing nightmare for her youngsters.

Strangely enough, the one person their mother was able to hide the seriousness of her problem from was their father. Either he didn't want to see it or he was too inebriated himself when they were together that he didn't recognize it. Either way, all he apparently cared about was having a loving drinking companion who took care of him as well as their children. He always made his wife feel like she was the responsible person in the family. And she knew she had to be, regardless of the pressure her husband put on her.

"I can't recall John ever complaining about how much I drank or what drugs I took," Dot used to say. "Maybe he really didn't want to know. We were drinking partners and we thought we were keeping it all very private—that is, until it got real bad.

"Once in a while when we would both wake up at the same time in the morning, I would ask my husband, 'How was I last night, honey? Did I act okay?' He would usually reply, 'You acted just fine, sweetheart. You didn't do anything out of the way. You were my sweet, loving girl.' Then he would hug me, swallow some pills, and get ready for the day."

Another reason Dot tried so hard to hide her problem was because many people still regarded alcoholics and drug addicts as the dregs of society. There was little or no understanding that alcoholism or chemical addiction was a disease. Most people thought it was evidence of a lack of willpower or low moral standards. Dot and her husband were always fearful that the world might possibly brand them as boozers and dope fiends. At this point in their lives, they truly believed they weren't. Yet, that fear didn't con-

vince them to change their lifestyle. It only made it more difficult to control.

As for the children, there was never a lack of material things.
They were well fed and clothed. They had toys, games, bicycles,
sports equipment, almost anything they might want or need.
They even had a pony and one of the first really big television sets
in town. In fact, many of their playmates envied them but were
also curious as to why they were seldom invited to play in the
Mooneys' house.

Still, as they grew older, there were enjoyable as well as disappointing times. During the summer, for example, John and
Dot would take them for a week's vacation to Tybee Beach, the
resort where they had spent their honeymoon. They would also
take Martha along to help. The boys would look forward to swimming in the surf all day with their parents and later going on rides
at the amusement park. But it rarely turned out that way.

The good doctor and his wife would send the children down to
the beach with Martha, promising to be along shortly. Then they
would have a drink to relax, and another and another, and never
make it to the beach or to the amusement park.

But it was different for a while during the Christmas sea-
son, when there was some real "family togetherness" and plenty
of holiday cheer. John had been retained for several years as a surgeon for the Central of Georgia Railway, in which capacity he
took care of employees who got sick or were injured in railroad
accidents. With the job came a family pass to ride the Central of
Georgia trains.

There was a special train called the Nancy Hanks that went
from Savannah through Statesboro and into Atlanta. About a
week or so before Christmas, John and the whole family would
hop aboard early in the morning and ride it into Atlanta. They
would have lunch and then have lots of laughs shopping for pres-
ents at Rich's Department Store until late in the afternoon. The
boys would have more fun playing on the train all the way back to

Statesboro. It was an annual family event until the railroad cancelled the physician's retainer.

John and Dot's oldest son, Al Mooney, who became a doctor like his father, as did his youngest brother, Bobby, today looks back at his childhood with a touch of sadness but also with a great deal of compassion and understanding.

"I've come to realize," he explained, "that all of the material things we were given were sort of a cover-up for the lack of depth in our relationship with our parents. It's not that they didn't love us. They were just having a great deal of difficulty with their addictions.

"It's funny, but I used to think my childhood was fine until I grew older and started thinking back. When you don't know anything else, I guess even chaos can seem normal.

"There was never any abuse," Al wanted to emphasize, "or neglect or abandonment, the kinds of things you hear about in some dysfunctional families. Even though you might have to say that our family was dysfunctional too at times, I think my folks did the best job they could under the circumstances.

"I do remember, however, that my brothers and I would often find ourselves in situations some people would not describe as normal. I guess I'd use the word 'confusing' because sometimes the explanations we'd be given for these situations by either my mother or my father just didn't make much sense."

For example, when Al and his brothers were very young and their parents would be going through a particularly argumentative period, Dot would drive them out to Jimps to stay with their grandparents for a few days. All the boys remember how much they enjoyed helping out on the farm, gathering eggs, milking cows, and being taken for a swim in the pond by their aunt Marilyn and uncle Arthur James. It was usually a fun time.

When things calmed down at Lee Street, Dot would come back out to take them home. Often she had been drinking. Al recalls one particularly harrowing event when he was about seven. His mother arrived at the farm late one afternoon more than a bit tipsy. At least that's what he heard his uncle Jim accuse her of rather loudly when he tried to take away her car keys. He said she was in no condition to drive and would be putting herself and the children in severe jeopardy.

Dot wouldn't listen. She got very angry, grabbed the keys back, ushered her sons into the car, and took off.

"Even though we were only six miles from Statesboro," Al remembered, "most of the drive was on a busy highway, Route 301. My mother was all over the road. I just sensed that she needed some help. So I stood in front of the car's dashboard clinging to the cold metal and peering through the windshield so that I could direct her."

His mother would swerve and her small son would shout, "No, Mom! Don't turn here! Turn off your blinkers! It's not time to turn yet!"

A moment later he would shout, "Stop going so fast! Get into the other lane, quick! There's a car trying to pass you!"

As Dot swerved into the right lane, her lack of control took her smack into a roadside ditch. The muddy ravine stopped the car from going any farther. Little Jimmy and Bobby, who were in the back seat, were thrown to the floor. Al hit his head against the windshield, receiving only a minor bump. Thank God no one was seriously hurt. However, when Dot saw that her sons were okay, she began yelling at Al for distracting her. Then, since they had only gone a few miles from Jimps, she told him to run back to his uncle's house and have him bring his tractor to pull them out of the ditch.

"It was already dark," the elder son recalled, "and I was scared to death I might get lost or get hit by a car. But I made it. By the time my uncle and I got back to my mother's car, she had already made up an excuse for the accident. Maybe it made sense to her but it made no sense at all to me or my uncle."

Dot told her brother that the highway department had been working on Route 301 and left some ruts of dirt in the right-hand lane. She said she hit one of the ruts, lost control, and that's how she landed in the ditch. The confusing explanations for bizarre behavior kept right on coming.

"At one point my dad was going away to more and more treatment places, sometimes for weeks at a time," Al continued. "He was still looking for a solution to his problem. My brothers and I never knew he had a problem then. We just thought he was acting very strange. But we were always curious when he wasn't around for a while."

On one of those first occasions when their father had been gone for a few days, his sons Al and Jimmy wanted to know where he was. So they asked their mother. "Oh, he's off learning how to be a better doctor," she replied.

"We thought that meant he was attending some medical thing and would be home shortly," Al said. "After a week or so, we asked our mother again and got the same reply, only this time in a more annoyed tone. We became really confused when our father suddenly began sending home newly made furniture, including some wooden toys and a toy trunk for us kids. When we asked where they came from, our mother simply said it was none of our business. A few years later we learned that our father had been in another treatment center and had been making furniture as part of his therapy. He laughed and said at least his woodworking hobby finally paid off."

It eventually became impossible for John and Dot to hide their erratic behavior from the rest of the family. As a result, relatives and close friends would compliment Al for being "the little man in the family" every time he handled another out-of-control situation.

These included scary and upsetting events like keeping his mother awake when she was driving with the children in the car or taking his brothers to their "Aunt Honey" and "Uncle Bill" Bowen's house a few doors away when all hell broke loose in his own home. The frightened young children would pick up their blankets and trudge across the yard in their pajamas, often staying there for days.

The Bowens, who remained friends with John and Dot through it all, became almost second parents to the Mooney boys during the worst part of their mother's and father's addiction. In fact, during the summer they would take the children to their beach house on St. Simons Island for weeks at a time to give them a respite from all the fights and bickering. Honey and Bill somehow realized they were dealing with two very sick but loving people who hopefully would someday find their way out of their morass and straighten out their lives.

As for Al Mooney, while he didn't come out of it unscathed, he says his survival brought him some important benefits: "I acquired a lot of self-confidence running rescue missions anytime the family train ran off the tracks. But at the age of ten, I shouldn't have been the engineer. I should have been just a kid playing in the backyard."

Jimmy Mooney grew up to be the businessman in the family, having graduated with a business degree from Georgia Southern University. He regrets, however, that as a child, he never had a very close relationship with his father. It took some years and some pain to bring that about.

"It seemed like my dad was always gone a lot," he explained. "At first it was his work as a physician. Back in those days, doctors made a lot of house calls and my father was no exception. Later on he wasn't around much because of the time he spent going on benders or in drying-out places, although I didn't know that at the time."

The one clear early recollection Jimmy has involving his father was riding up front with him in his brand-new white 1956 Thunderbird Classic convertible. He was about six years old at the time.

"My dad was so proud of that car and I was so proud to be sitting right next to him when he took it for a ride shortly after buying it. I found out that he actually went up to Detroit to watch them put the finishing touches to that car and then drove it all the way back to Statesboro. I think that white Thunderbird helped pump up his ego quite a bit."

When asked if he thought his father could really afford such an expensive luxury automobile at that time in his life, Jimmy smiled and replied, "It didn't matter to my father if he was doing well financially or not. If he wanted something, he went out and got it and let the other bills wait. That's why at one point we had an unpaid five-hundred-dollar milk bill and owed the electric company and many others too."

Jimmy went on to explain that it was his mom who really raised him and his brothers, "and boy, was she a strict disciplinarian, especially when she was sober. We could always tell the difference in the way she was.

"Things were usually unpredictable at our house. She would whip us sometimes just because we were noisy, so I stopped being noisy. But with three little boys running around the house and her with a hangover, I can now understand why she would get out of sorts. I didn't know then that it was the alcohol and drugs that made her unpredictable. After she hit us, she would feel guilty. She'd kiss us and hug us and tell us how sorry she was—until the next time.

"In spite of it all, she was really a very loving mother. I felt pretty close to her and always knew that she loved me. She tried so hard to take good care of us, even becoming a den mother for the Cub Scouts for a while. But because of what she was doing to herself, she had a hard time dealing with her emotions. I just didn't know it at the time."

One of Jimmy's earliest recollections involving his mother was the day he had his first beer. He was around four or five years old. Dot would often take him and his brothers out to visit her family on weekends. The relatives would gather and there would usually be a party.

He remembers one particular weekend going with his uncles and cousins down to the big pond where they went swimming.

He watched them catch a whole bunch of catfish, which they brought back to the Riggses' farmhouse for a big fish fry.

"There was always drinking that went along with these things," Jimmy continued. "I can remember sitting next to my mother and her giving me a beer to drink. I didn't like it at all. I don't have the best memory in the world, but I can still recall how that beer tasted and I didn't like it one bit. I thought to myself, why do people drink that stuff?"

Strangely enough, Jimmy Mooney later became an alcoholic himself and had a lot of his own troubles to deal with. Today he has recovered from the disease of alcoholism and leads a very successful and sober life while helping others to do the same.

Even though he was the baby of the family at that time, Bobby Mooney didn't escape his mother's wrath nor did he escape her love: "I recall the mornings she would have trouble getting out of bed. I didn't know why. I just thought she was tired. I was maybe two or three at the time and I would manage to climb in next to her and she would snuggle me close and tickle me. She would give me all the love and affection she could. I loved my mother and I know that she loved me.

"But there were also those times when I got a little older and would get my ass whipped real good and wonder why. Of course there were many more occasions when I got it whipped and knew exactly why."

One of those occasions involved a snake, a little green critter that Bobby, who was about four at the time, planned to grow into a big green critter. Only his mother, who hated snakes, found the can he was raising it in near the back door and threw the can and the critter away.

"When I asked if she had seen my snake," he recalled, "my mother didn't admit to a thing. But I pretty much knew she was lying about it and I got mad. There was a case of empty Coca-Cola bottles in the backyard. I was so angry I started breaking them against a brick wall near the house. My mother came storming out and spanked my little butt nearly clean off. I had to admit I deserved it but wouldn't tell her that."

Bobby also remembered that every year his mother took him and his brothers and sometimes a few of their friends on a camping trip to a place called Tallulah River. Once in a while their aunt Marilyn would come along.

Bobby described their mode of transportation to the campsite: "My father had his Thunderbird and my mom had this big old station wagon that seemed as if it could carry a zillion people. It would be dragging on the ground it would be so full of kids sometimes. My mother loved kids. We would go up there to the mountains and roam through the woods for two weeks at a time. My dad rarely came. My mother used to say he was always too busy."

As for the things he did with his father as a child, Bobby has vague memories of being with John in his darkroom upstairs in his home, watching him work at his brand-new photography hobby: "I just remember how it seemed like magic. He would do a print in the enlarger, put it into the development solution, and slowly a picture would appear. It was fascinating—so fascinating in fact that I got into photography myself and I still love it after all these years."

As for the war, while Bobby doesn't remember most of what was said at the time, he does recall with some emotion sitting in his father's lap as a child listening to him talk about his experiences on the battlefield. He would then show his little boy things he had brought home from the fighting—a German swastika, a German Luger, some empty shells, and pictures of his field hospital with his medical team standing outside.

Again, being so little, the youngest Mooney son was also confused by his parents' behavior but had no idea at the time it had anything to do with alcohol and drugs. And, ironically enough, Bobby, like his brother Jimmy, also became an alcoholic some years later and today is recovered and helping others find sobriety.

When John returned from another hospital or institution, he would usually remain fairly clean and sober for a short period of time. Although he was continuing to live a lie that many people around him were beginning to see right through, he did his best to maintain the appearance of temperance and respectability. This was especially true at the hospital, his medical practice, and at the places he most often frequented in Statesboro. But it was becoming an immense struggle.

During his more or less sober periods, John and Dot would try to maintain a semblance of normality. They would go dancing, attend parties, and socialize with old friends. But they would always try to leave before they became too tipsy, fearful of exposing themselves. While Dot did her level best, she wasn't always as successful as her husband. By now she had to fortify herself in order to face what she considered social pressures. Neither one of them knew how things would turn out on those evenings.

"Sometimes I would wake up the next morning and discover that my nightgown was on backwards," she once laughingly told a close friend. "That's when I knew I had gotten home so drunk that John had to undress me and put me to bed. But he never would say a word about it. He saved it and used it as ammunition for our next argument."

And by now there was always a next argument. Sometimes one would break out over the simplest, most foolish thing. For example, one night the children were watching television with their parents in the living room. Dot had Bobby in her arms, and Al and Jimmy were seated next to their father. They were both now in school and needed their sleep. It was past their bedtime, so she told them to kiss their father goodnight and follow her upstairs.

John looked at her rather sternly and said, "No, this is an educational program. Why don't they stay down here and watch the rest of the show with us?"

Since she was trying to enforce a few rules for the children and didn't like to be contradicted, Dot replied rather sarcastically,

"Well, honey, since you're so much wiser and better educated than I am, I guess you know best. I'm just trying to make sure the boys get enough rest for school."

Annoyed by her tone, her husband replied, "You're right. You're their mother. I'm only their father. You run things around here. They need to go right to bed."

Little Al and Jimmy, trying to take advantage of the situation, had moved a little closer to their father, which bothered Dot all the more.

"No, you put them to bed whenever you're good and ready," she replied. Then she turned and headed upstairs with Bobby in her arms. John got up and followed, saying, "I said you were right. What more do you want from me?"

The argument went on for more than an hour, keeping all three of their sons wide awake. As Dot later explained, "Our continued drinking and drugging only made things worse. Sometimes we'd come home from a party and wind up screaming and yelling at each other until two or three o'clock in the morning. I used to hate it when he would tell me how superior he was because he was a doctor and had more education than I did. I'd yell back that I had more common sense and wouldn't be ruining everything I worked for." Their arguments often woke up the children and their neighbors, but they would keep on fighting anyway.

"I remember one particular night," Al Mooney recalls, "lying at the top of the stairs listening to a really physical argument that finally came to blows. I was maybe seven or eight. I remember lying there and listening for hours and just being really confused and frightened about what was going on."

Sometimes his parents were already undressed for bed when an argument broke out. John would be in his pajamas and his wife in a thin negligee. One would follow the other into the bar area in the living room to get another drink, both of them yelling all the way. In order to end some arguments, Dot would shout at her husband: "If you think I'm going to put up with this anymore, you're crazy! I'm taking the car and getting out of here!"

Then they would fight over the car keys all the way to the front door. If Dot won, she would stagger out into the street in her negligee and bare feet, slide into the car, and screech away from the curb. At first she thought she did it because it really bothered her husband. She knew how concerned he would be that she might pass out and crash the car, or wind up in a blackout and get lost somewhere. Dot was soon to discover for herself why she really did it. She was beginning to have suicidal tendencies.

If John won the battle for the car keys, he would often just take her into his arms, hold her tight until she stopped pulling away, and blubber an apology. After a few moments, they would stagger back into their bedroom and fall into bed in each other's arms.

Dot found that her car came in handy whenever she couldn't sleep and needed her drugs. She had a terrible fear of her husband discovering she was taking so many heavy narcotics; she worried that he might waken while she was doing it in the house. So she would sneak out of their bedroom and head outside to the car to get her fix.

"The only problem was," she once said, "my car door squeaked rather loudly when you opened it. I always meant to oil it but never got around to it. Also, the light inside the car would come on and I'd worry about John or somebody seeing me in there."

One night when she had run out of her own drugs, she found a bottle of Demerol in a small cabinet under her kitchen counter. She went out to the car, took one shot of the Demerol out of a 30 cc vial and went back to bed. She still couldn't sleep. So she went back out and took another shot, then later another and another.

"I didn't realize it until sometime later," she continued, "that I had made fifteen trips to my car that night and into the early morning hours and took fifteen shots of Demerol. I could have overdosed. God certainly was with me."

The next day the problem continued.

"My husband called me from his office," she said, "and told me he had misplaced a bottle of Demerol somewhere and wondered if I had seen it. I was still in such a fog that I didn't know what to say. I simply told him I would look around for it and call him back.

"Now, talk about insanity. I actually went out into the yard, gazed all around, and even opened the garbage can to see what was in it. It wasn't until I came back into the kitchen and glanced at that cabinet that I suddenly realized what I had done. My hands were trembling when I called my husband back and told him I couldn't find any bottle of Demerol. That was only one of the many lies I told to cover up my addiction."

In the midst of her struggle to regain some kind of control over the amount of alcohol and sedatives she was consuming, Dot received word late one afternoon that only made things terribly more difficult to handle. Arthur Riggs, the father she loved and had disappointed so many times, had passed away.

Dot was high when she got the news and even higher when she attended the funeral. After it was over, her brother Jim told her how ashamed he was of her and that he would rather not see her at all than to see her in such a state. Every time she went to visit her mother after her father's death, she would always feel guilty for not being there when he was very sick. Myrtis tried to console her daughter but she couldn't keep her sober. Dot never forgave herself until some years later when she finally found a whole new way to live her life.

Meanwhile, John was continuing to make the rounds of more and more hospitals and psychiatric institutions. He was being diagnosed as having all kinds of mental ailments. This only convinced him even more that he drank and drugged because he was crazy, not an alcoholic or drug addict. In other words, he would rather be crazy so long as he could take something to keep himself sane. Of course, that reasoning only made sense to a real addict.

"Just about every time I was diagnosed," the very sick physician once explained, "my brain and my body were saturated with addictive substances. My brain was never clean. Yet these so-called specialists still believed what they were telling me, and so did I.

"I was told by one psychiatrist I had schizophrenia. Another said I was manic-depressive and also had psychoneurosis. One even said I was a constitutional psychopath, which meant I was born crazy and there was nothing I could do about it. That diagnosis gave me all the excuses I needed to keep pouring all that stuff into me. On top of it, those doctors prescribed even more stuff for me to pour in."

At one rehabilitation hospital in Savannah, John was given shots that did little to relieve his stress and tension. One day a lovely little nurse's aide came into his room and smiled. "Let me give you a good rubdown," she said, "and you'll feel a whole lot better."

Halfway through the rubdown, a bell rang and the pretty little aide had to leave to care for another patient. The physician sat up and noticed she had left the bottle of rubbing alcohol on his bedside table.

"I remember reading the label," he once shared, "and the warning about it causing serious gastric disturbances. By golly, I just didn't believe it. I poured out a glassful and drank it. It didn't cause any real serious gastric problems. From then on, whenever the going became difficult and money was in short supply, I drank rubbing alcohol."

John's finances were completely out of control. Money was indeed in very short supply, mainly because the income from his medical practice was rapidly dwindling. Many of his patients were getting fed up with his frequent absences, often for weeks at a time, and were going to see other doctors.

He owed large sums to grocers, druggists, gas stations, the electric company, more than five hundred dollars to the milk company, and three years of back taxes to the Internal Revenue Service. In an attempt to keep abreast of his overdue bills, he used his large home on Lee Street like an ATM machine. He periodically remortgaged the house and paid off what he could. Then, when he became delinquent again, he would borrow once more.

By 1957, the ATM stopped working. John had built his home in 1937 at the cost of $7,500. Now, twenty years later, he found there was no longer any equity left.

It was around this time that the practically bankrupt physician found a certified public accountant in town he came to rely on. His name was Earl Dabbs. John had delivered Earl's three children a few years earlier. Although Earl was twenty years younger, he had known Dr. Mooney as a teenager. He had gone off to college and after graduation had joined the IRS for a few years. He left to return to Statesboro and opened his own CPA firm. He was now a skilled financial expert and a respected businessman around town.

"I had always thought that Dr. Mooney was a super-smart, highly intelligent man as well as a great doctor," Earl said of the person he would not only come to help survive great adversity but also help achieve admired and heralded success. "However, I must say that he was not a good manager of money. The more we got to know each other, the more I came to realize that for John, money was something to be spent, not saved and accumulated. And he often spent it before he had it."

When asked how the financially strapped physician and his family were able to survive during the late 1950s when everything was crashing in on them, Dr. Mooney's trusted accountant replied, "John had some very good friends in town that he could always call on to endorse his notes, men who never lost faith in him. I think we could all see that he was a very good and decent man who had serious problems and we just wanted to help him.

"Ike Minkovitz was one of them. Ike was a kind, Jewish businessman who owned a big department store in town. He was also a real saver who had great credit. He was a good man who liked and respected John Mooney so much that he was always willing to endorse a note for him, right to the very end. Bill Bowen, our mayor, was another one. And Gus Sawyer, who was in the insurance business. They all thought the world of John. And especially

Professor Jack Averitt, who I believe saved John's life back in 1959. He loved John and was willing to do anything to help him.

"Even his attorney, George Johnston, never lost faith even though, like almost everyone else in town, we knew he drank too much and took drugs. But we also knew that he always took great care in treating his patients.

"I remember one day after he had finally sobered up he said to me that one of the proudest moments of his life was when he walked into a bank and borrowed some money without anyone having to endorse his note."

Earl said he had heard stories about his friend admitting people to Bulloch County Hospital, performing surgery on them, and then going on a bender for a few days. He said the patients would complain about the difficulty of getting out of the hospital but never complained about the surgery.

"He was that good a doctor, but that's how he would lose patients and lose income at the same time," the accountant said. "Fortunately he had a great nurse working for him named Dallas Cason. She was able to pull his bacon out of the fire for a number of years."

What Earl Dabbs said about Dallas Cason was absolutely true. However, Dallas said that when she first went to work for Dr. Mooney, she never saw him the least bit tipsy when he came into the office after performing surgery at the hospital, nor did he drink while treating his patients.

"His problem was something that evolved over time," she explained. "But for quite awhile, despite his growing number of absences from his practice due to his drinking and drugging and going places to dry out, he was the perfect doctor. He taught me how to use our new X-ray machine, make casts after he would set bone fractures, and to assist him with minor surgery like sewing up severe lacerations or removing tonsils.

"I also learned his way of keeping good medical charts on

patients, taking blood pressures and giving shots. We did all these things in the office and he was excellent with patients. That's why they loved and respected him so much."

That's also why the dedicated nurse was so surprised when Dr. Mooney started going on benders. Then she had another surprise not long after she started her new job. She found she was pregnant with her third child.

"I thought the only thing I could do was to hand in my resignation," Dallas said, "mainly because I wanted to nurse this baby. Dot came to me and said I mustn't leave, that her husband needed me and that she would help take care of the child while I continued working.

"As I said, Dot and I had developed such a good relationship by this time, and Dr. John kept saying how much he depended upon me that I agreed to stay. In fact, I worked right up until a few weeks before my son was born."

The nurse stayed home for about a month after giving birth while an RN from the hospital temporarily replaced her. Then she came back to the medical office, baby and all. Dot kept her promise. She was there every day caring for the infant while Dallas assisted her husband. When the child was a little more than four months old, the nurse's mother-in-law took the baby into her house and cared for him together with the twins. Dallas spent more and more of her time watching over her impaired physician.

Ironically, the young nurse's husband, Jay, wasn't much help at home because he too was drinking heavily. However, since he continued to work, take care of their house, and bring in a paycheck, he too denied he was an alcoholic for a number of years. And since Dallas herself knew little about the disease of addiction at that time, she just hoped that something would happen one day and both her husband and her boss would simply stop.

"As for the Mooney family," she said, "we all became very close. We didn't socialize but we became the very best of friends. And as their problems increased because of their addictions, I tried to be there for them. My daddy used to tell me that if you can't be a friend when someone really needs you, you're not really a friend at all."

She recalled the time when Jimmy Mooney was born and required intestinal surgery. Dallas stayed with him at the hospital for several hours each evening to give his parents time to at least have dinner together.

"Dot was very attentive to her children before things got really bad," she explained. "She loved those kids so much and would go places with them and do things. So she was beside herself when little Jimmy needed that surgery. She stayed with him at the hospital all day and was exhausted by the evening. So, since my mother-in-law didn't mind, I would go and watch over Jimmy so Dot and her husband could have a little break. And yes, I could always tell they had been drinking quite a bit when they returned. But that was none of my business."

In fact, Dallas never talked to her boss about his imbibing, even when it became very noticeable or when he would go on benders or, later, to drying-out places. That's when she would make up stories to cover his sudden disappearances. There were other times the physician would let her off the hook by making up his own stories in advance. Several times when he was getting ready to check into another institution, he prepared the way himself by putting notices in the local newspapers. One notice might say, for example, that he was going to be away for several weeks studying an important new surgical breakthrough at some leading medical center. Another might report that he was on sabbatical to investigate the latest cures for some new viral diseases and still another that he was taking a four-week graduate course in orthopedic surgery in California. Drunk or sober, Dr. John Mooney was quite creative.

"Since I never felt very good about making up stories myself," the loyal nurse said, smiling, "when he did it himself, I was grateful—or as grateful as one could be under those kinds of circumstances.

"When he returned sober, he might simply say that he enjoyed his time in the mountains getting straightened out or would laugh and say that one more psychiatrist told him he was a mental case, not an alcoholic."

By 1957, Dr. John Mooney wasn't the only one going to see psychiatrists. Dot Mooney herself was now searching for answers. Her "spells" were getting worse, her relationship with her husband was rapidly deteriorating, and her ability to care for her children was growing more difficult by the day.

"I found someone I thought was a wonderful psychiatrist in Savannah," Dot once explained, "but practically every time I went to see him, he gave me a different pill. He never took any away from me, and I had plenty of different pills at home. I really didn't need any more. Still, he'd give me a new pill during almost every visit.

"I remember he once asked me if I drank a lot. I told him I had an occasional drink with my husband and, for a moment, I almost believed it. I know I wanted to believe it because I didn't want my drinking and my drugging to be my real problem. I found out later, that's a form of denial. I had the kind of illness that kept telling me I didn't have an illness.

"Denial can sometimes be so strong that no matter what you say or what you feel or how bad you hurt, it's going to tell you you're not really an addict."

One day she admitted to her psychiatrist that she drank more than she had initially told him. He said he had known she was lying. Then she asked why he thought that, even after taking all these pills, she still drank so much. As he began to probe more deeply into her background, Dot suddenly remembered her mother once telling her she had some Lumbee Indian blood coursing through her veins. Maybe that's the problem, she thought, since she had heard so many stories about American Indians drinking too much firewater—that they were prone to having a serious problem with alcohol.

She did some checking into the Lumbee tribe, descendants of

the Siouan- and Algonquian-speaking Cheraw Indians, and discovered that many of them had intermarried with white, black, and Cherokee people. While she couldn't directly trace her own ancestry, her mother's comments were all Dot needed to convince her that American Indian blood in her veins posed an irreversible part of her problem. It was one more avenue she had gone down that led to another dead end. And her doctor wasn't giving her any of the answers she was looking for—answers she desperately wanted that could lead her out of her terrible dilemma.

"So I started threatening him like I was doing with practically everyone in my life at this point," the now almost hopeless wife and mother shared. "I told him that if he couldn't do something for me, that if he couldn't help me feel better and stop doing all the terrible things I was doing, that I was going to kill myself."

Since the psychiatrist had already diagnosed his patient with severe depression and suicidal tendencies, he decided to take a drastic step—one that had been very controversial in the medical profession for many years.

He started Dot Mooney on electric shock treatments.

CHAPTER EIGHT

No End in Sight

THEY ONCE CALLED IT A "GEORGIA POWER COCKTAIL"—THE practice of attaching electrodes to the scalp of a mentally troubled patient and jolting the patient's brain with an electrical current until the subject went into convulsions.

Today medical science calls it "electroconvulsive therapy," or ECT. Most people still refer to it as electric shock therapy. When first pioneered in the 1930s, it was a crude and frightening practice that often left patients dazed and disoriented, and some of them even dead. Yet its use in treating everything from depression to mania to schizophrenia quickly spread far and wide until influential voices in the field of mental health began to challenge its efficacy.

As a result of attacks on psychiatrists and others using the procedure, electric shock therapy waned over the years and almost vanished entirely from the psychiatric scene by the end of the 1960s. Also, the successful 1975 movie *One Flew Over the Cuckoo's Nest,* in which Jack Nicholson's character received unnecessary shock treatments, played a major role in further discrediting ECT.

At the same time, powerful new drugs had been developed in the interim that offered alternative treatments for a wide variety of mental problems. These new psychotropic medications were very much welcomed since they were not nearly as barbaric as jolting a patient with an electrical current that could produce a grand mal seizure.

However, ECT never completely disappeared as a last-resort treatment, as many people may still think. Instead, it gradually began making a comeback.

Some countries actually passed laws to ban it. Others, such as Canada, Germany, Japan, China, the Netherlands, and Austria, greatly restricted its use. But in the United States, more than 100,000 people—two-thirds of them women—receive electric shock therapy treatments every year. And, as of 2011, according to the American Psychiatric Association, those numbers are increasing.

Some leading researchers in the mental health field have made extraordinary claims that ECT actually causes brain cells to be renewed, not destroyed as once thought—that electric shock therapy promotes the development of new nerve cells in the brain that are involved with memory and emotion, thus helping severely depressed and mentally challenged patients.

At the same time, there is a very good reason why ECT has been so demonized and created such a high level of distrust among many psychiatrists. To this day, no one has been able to adequately explain what goes on when 220 volts of electricity zip through the brain. The only reason grand mal seizures and deaths are rare these days, claim its detractors, is the drugs that are now used to relax and anesthetize patients prior to treatments.

Despite all the criticisms, many psychiatrists still believe that modern versions of ECT offer the last, best hope for patients suffering intractable psychiatric disorders.

The primary drug used with most electric shock therapy is Sodium Pentothal, also known as "truth serum" as a result of numerous films about FBI investigations and spies. It is a tranquilizer that, given in small doses before treatment, relieves tension and anxiety and creates an almost dreamlike feeling. That could have been the reason why Dot Mooney fell in love with electric shock therapy.

"I heard many people say how horrible it was," she once admitted. "That's why I didn't say a word to anybody for a long time that I not only had shock treatments but that I also loved them. I became addicted to them. But I didn't want people to think I was strange."

In the beginning, her psychiatrist was giving Dot two or three treatments a week. But if she felt a "nervous spell" coming on, she would call him up, jump in her car, and head for Savannah for another treatment.

"They gave me Sodium Pentothal," she said, "and it didn't take me very long to become addicted to it. Just put that Sodium Pentothal into my vein and I drifted off to the most pleasant places you could imagine. And then it became total oblivion, exactly what I was looking for."

She didn't mind the electrodes pressed against her scalp or the ominous hum of the electrical equipment surrounding her. She didn't even mind the sound of the shocking sensation she would describe as "zzzz" or "kzzz" that zipped through her brain. Dot Mooney wanted relief, and Sodium Pentothal and a brief electrical current gave it to her.

"I didn't care about anything," Dot once shared openly and honestly with some very close friends. "I just wanted to stop this mind of mine from driving me crazy with everything running through it. And this was the only relief I thought I had at this point. Dear God, I would have taken that drug every four hours if they would have given it to me."

The desperate mother of three claimed that electric shock treatments and Sodium Pentothal kept her alive and sane until she was finally able to find her way out of the hell she was in.

"I can't say that I was really grateful for it," she explained, "but I don't resent going through it. That was absolutely the craziest and most frustrating period of my life. What I am grateful for is that I came out of it alive and with a fairly reasonable mental capacity."

While Dot Mooney believed electric shock treatments were of significant benefit to her, she was far less enthusiastic when it came to its application to others, particularly her husband.

Dallas Cason remembers the day Dot dropped by the office to pick up some of her medical records she needed to give to her psychiatrist. She broke down and told the nurse she had decided to try electric shock therapy to help alleviate her spells and depression. Dallas was quite taken aback since she knew little about ECT, only the horror stories.

Her concern grew somewhat intense, however, when her boss's wife mentioned that her psychiatrist thought Dr. Mooney might also be an excellent candidate for the controversial therapy. She was much relieved when Dot remarked, "While I have a lot of confidence in this psychiatrist, I've heard others say some people don't always get their brains working normally again after a number of treatments. I'm not so worried about myself, but I would never want John to take a chance. If electrical shock therapy somehow affected his brain, he might never be able to work again."

Dallas said she totally agreed. It also made her realize how much Dot Mooney still loved her husband and cared for his welfare despite the constantly growing disruptions in their lives that she couldn't always understand or was unable or unwilling to do anything about. The subject of Dr. Mooney and ECT, however, never came up again.

It was now late summer of 1957. The Mooney boys were at St. Simons Island with the Bowens. Dot was in Savannah having another electrical fix for her "nervous spells." John was sitting all alone in his living room at Lee Street, nursing a bottle of Scotch. He was trying to ignore the fact that life was closing in on him with no end in sight for all his difficulties. As he slowly drank his way into another stupor, little did he know he was about to be offered the real answer to all his problems once again.

The front doorbell rang. The half-inebriated physician hesitated a moment, then went to the door and opened it. In stepped his old friend Henry, whom he hadn't seen in a long, long time. He and Henry had grown up together but had since gone their separate ways.

"I had known Henry all my life," John said as he once recalled that particular afternoon. "I had watched this poor fella throw himself away with alcohol, and I just felt so sorry for him. I'd seen him rise to be a high-ranking officer in the army, an owner of a very prosperous business, and then watched the poor fella just continue to drink until he lost everything and landed in the gutter.

"I thought at first he was coming to see me for a handout. But when I saw how good he looked and how well he was dressed, I got a little confused. Then I discovered he was coming to talk to me, and what he said caught me a bit off guard."

After some brief comments about the weather and some gossip going around town, John's slightly nervous friend said that he had finally found sobriety through the program of Alcoholics Anonymous and was now doing quite well. He said he was a member of the Statesboro AA group.

"I remember thinking to myself," the physician said, "boy, this is wonderful. This fella has really come out of the gutter to amount to something. Then Henry asked me if I would like to go to an AA meeting with him some night."

With his usual arrogance and self-denial, John replied, "I sure would, Henry. I know a lot about that addiction stuff. You get your fellas together and I'll come down to your group some night and tell you all about alcoholism any time you want me to."

The drunken doctor had no idea that his friend was making what they term in Alcoholics Anonymous "a Twelve-Step call" on him. That's when one or more sober members of the AA program go to see someone suffering from the disease of alcoholism in hopes of helping them find sobriety. But this time, Henry was up against a seemingly hopeless case.

"I'll never forget the look on poor Henry's face as he left," John said. "He was shaking his head. I guess he went back to his group and waited for me to die. He knew the truth, that I had too much pride, too big an ego, and a very closed mind. I had this almost innate refusal to see myself as I was at any cost and it wasn't going to get any better until something happened—something that could crack open the shell I had built around myself.

"And I wouldn't let anybody have a peep inside that shell. You see, while I tried to portray this phony image of myself as somebody special, I really didn't have a very good opinion of the guy inside the shell."

After Henry left, the tortured physician sat staring at his bottle of Scotch. He knew deep inside that when you have so much false pride, you come to resent the people who are trying to help you. In your mixed-up mind, you accuse them of trying to do something to you rather than doing something for you.

"When you get into this kind of mind-set," the physician once explained, "there's no way even God can get through to you. While I never lost my belief in God, I often wondered if He wanted anything more to do with me.

"When you still feel you're something special and regard yourself as a prominent physician rather than the alcoholic and drug addict you really are, something really bad is sure to happen."

By the spring of 1958, the really bad part was already starting to happen.

Perhaps the one thing Dr. John Mooney prized most in his life was his surgical skill. He had established a reputation as one of the finest surgeons in the South. He was often called on to consult with other surgeons on difficult cases. Now, each time he would enter the operating room, he was fearful that he might not be able to perform up to his own high standards. It showed in his eyes. It showed in the perspiration on his brow and sometimes in the barely perceptible tremble in his hands.

Other doctors at Bulloch County Hospital were beginning to take notice. A few began backing away from working with John. His real friends, however, stood by and tried to help without causing him any obvious embarrassment.

John would start scrubbing up for surgery and then happen to see one of his friends scrubbing up nearby. When he would glance over, his fellow doctor might say, "I heard you have an interesting case this morning, John. Do you mind if I observe? There's still a whole lot I can learn."

Some less diplomatic doctors would look at him and comment to each other, "Hey, John's all right this morning. We won't have to scrub up with him."

Recalling those times, John once said, "At first I'd get mad. I'd think, who needs them? I can operate by myself. I don't require any help from any well-meaning colleagues. But gradually, as I began to question my own judgment, I came to appreciate them being there for me.

"I was becoming more and more concerned about possibly making a mistake and if I did, I'd have help correcting it. Many doctors make mistakes, usually very minor ones and easily correctable. With me, I had a reason to worry about it. I think it only happened once or twice, and nothing very serious. I was always determined to be in control in the operating room. When I didn't think I could be, I usually cancelled the surgery or had another surgeon handle the case for me."

John's close friend Dr. Bird Daniel once explained things this way: "You don't throw away surgeons like John Mooney in a small community like ours. Sometimes I would postpone whatever procedure we had scheduled to do together until I had gotten a gallon or so of coffee into him. Not that he ever came in roaring drunk. That wasn't his way.

"But the effects of the chemicals he was pouring into his body never fully left him. At first he got mad as a wet tomcat when I scrubbed in with him one morning, but I think he realized it was just a precaution. His technique was always first class, and I never once had to take the knife out of his hands."

What Dr. Daniel didn't say was that he was sorely tempted to do so on more than one occasion. And it bothered him greatly to watch his dear friend and associate continue spiraling downward in his addictions. Yet, every time he broached the subject, he was politely silenced. So he stopped even alluding to the problem and just went on praying and standing by his friend and fellow surgeon.

Around the middle of the summer of 1958, things got so bad in the Mooney household that Dot went to her husband and begged that they make another serious attempt at getting off alcohol and drugs for good. While she was still going for her electric shock treatments, her addiction to Sodium Pentothal had become so intense that few other drugs could satisfy her craving. Also, in her moments of clarity, she could see her husband's medical practice disintegrating before his eyes, his health worsening, and her children not knowing where to turn for comfort and support.

John agreed. So once again the boys were sent off to their grandmother's house in Jimps while their parents left to engage in one more battle with their addictions.

In his many previous travels to find recovery, the physician had heard of a psychiatric facility in Asheville, North Carolina, where he believed they could be detoxed in a week or so from all the sedatives in their systems. John and Dot truly believed they could make a brand-new start. It's like that for most addicts in denial—they believe that once their brains are rid of all booze and drugs, they can stay clean and sober on their own.

When the couple arrived in Asheville, they discovered the hospital would not accept them as patients unless they agreed to stay for the entire eight-week recovery program.

"There's no way we can stay that long," John said to Dot. "The most time I can spare from my practice is two weeks. I've been losing too many patients as it is."

Seeing the disappointed, almost hopeless look on his wife's face,

John came up with another idea. Since he was a doctor and she was a nurse, they knew how to detox people from alcohol and drugs. Therefore, they should be able to safely give each other a life-threatening treatment called insulin shock therapy and detox themselves.

While she was a bit hesitant, Dot knew that her husband was an excellent and experienced physician. She still had faith in him and, perhaps even more important, she was desperate to get off everything she was continuing to ingest.

So, after she agreed to her husband's plan to clean out all the narcotics in their bodies and in their brains, they went shopping. He bought all the necessary medical supplies, including glucose, orange juice, syringes, and a sterilizer. Then they checked into a small, cheap motel on the outskirts of town.

The physician arranged his purchases on a cigarette-scarred bureau. Dot turned down the covers on the two double beds in the hot, muggy room. Then her husband started the procedure that would hopefully break the habit that had had them in its clutches for far too many years.

Coming off drugs is a terrible ordeal even under the best of circumstances. During the first seven days in that dingy motel room, there were times when John Mooney lay in ashen shock on his damp mattress. And there were times when Dot would lapse into a coma, her skin warm and clammy. Sometimes they would both lie there moaning in a semiconscious state, wondering how much more they could possibly endure. "I don't know any reason for our not dying in that room other than the fact that a loving God had some other plans for us," John once admitted.

By the end of the next seven days, they were both so sick and weak that they had to call for an ambulance to take them back to Statesboro, where they recovered at Bulloch Hospital. They also had to hire a man from Asheville to follow them back in their car. By the end of the third seven days, they were both drinking and drugging again.

Recalling that experience of detoxing in that motel room, Dot said, "I used to try and make myself feel better by saying the drugs I took didn't come off the street. I got them from legal prescriptions. Still, my stomach and my mind didn't know the difference. They reacted the same way and got me into the same kind of trouble that street drugs do.

"Even though I could have died in that motel room, it didn't frighten me enough to stop. I don't believe you can really scare alcoholics and drug addicts into stopping. For example, I also went right back to my electric shock treatments despite the things I heard people say about the danger involved. I guess when you want to escape your problems, you'll do almost anything."

Her husband put it another way: "We were both in awful shape after what we tried, and neither of us was very proud of the shape the other was in. But we went on. What else can you do but go on until you finally reach the end of the line. And I knew that for me, the end of the line was fast approaching."

What remained of John's once lucrative medical practice was being held together by his loyal and trusted nurse. The deep and unwavering friendship that Dallas Cason exhibited toward John and Dot Mooney went far beyond what anyone could imagine.

For example, because of the physician's frequent absences from the office and Dot's growing inability to manage things at home, Dallas was now handling most of the financial transactions for the medical practice. She was paying the bills and collecting payments, as well as handling more and more of the various patient treatments.

"Thank goodness there were quite a few uncollected bills on the books," the nurse explained. "I kept hoping they were still collectable. They were there mainly because Dr. Mooney never wanted to pressure his patients into paying, particularly when they had some financial difficulties of their own. Maybe that's one reason why patients were still coming to see him, although I must confess, even in the face of what was going on, a whole lot of people still believed in him. He was their doctor no matter what."

Dallas said the physician also owed a lot of money around town, much of it to local drugstores. And they wanted to be paid for all the prescription drugs he was ordering.

"I would dole out these payments as best I could, attempting to keep everyone happy," she said. "There were some days I don't know how Dr. Mooney managed to keep things going. Surprisingly there was always enough to cover my pay. He made sure of that."

The nurse believed the doctor kept things afloat by borrowing from everyone he could as well as using whatever equity he had left in his home. She was stunned by how much money he was going through on things she knew little about. However, despite her suspicions, she never questioned him. She admits she really didn't want to know.

At times the financial pressure on the practice grew so intense that Dallas would get in her car and drive to patients' homes in the area in an attempt to collect long-overdue bills.

"I remember one day, all I came back with was a car full of chickens," she said, with a slight grimace. "Fortunately, a local grocer took them off my hands for a few dollars."

Since the nurse's relationship with John and Dot had become so close and personal, she was now being called to the Mooney home when matters got out of control. There were times she arrived at Lee Street only to find the police already there, doing their best to calm things down. She would find the children huddled up on the staircase crying, Martha trying to force some coffee into Dot, and the police sergeant who had known the inebriated physician all his life threatening to arrest him if he didn't do what he was told.

Sometimes Dallas would ask her husband, Jay, to accompany her because he and John had become good friends too and he just might help smooth things over. Also, she hoped that seeing such a fracas might influence Jay to stop drinking himself. It never did.

There was one particular weekend that Dallas Cason would never forget: "It was about eleven on a Saturday night. I was just going to bed when the phone rang. It was Honey Bowen. She sounded real upset. She told me she and Bill had taken the boys to their house because Dr. Mooney and his wife were terribly drunk. They were screaming at each other and throwing things around. She was afraid one of the neighbors might call the police again and this time they could cart John right off to jail.

"Honey begged me to come right over. For some reason she felt I could talk to them at times like this. My husband was fairly sober that night so I convinced him to drive me over to Statesboro."

It was a scene from *Who's Afraid of Virginia Woolf?* John was downstairs, very intoxicated and roaming through the house in his underwear. He was carrying a shotgun and yelling incoherently at his wife, who was upstairs trying to crawl out a window onto the roof. Dallas and her husband could hear her screaming for help.

"Of course I was shocked and frightened when I walked into the house and saw Dr. Mooney waving that shotgun all around," the nurse said. "I had never known him to be the least bit violent or abusive to anyone, not since the day we met. And now to see this. I just couldn't believe my eyes. Neither could my husband.

"We didn't know at first whether he was thinking of shooting Dot or shooting himself or even shooting anyone who walked into the house. We didn't even know if the gun was loaded, which, thank God, we found out later it wasn't. But he was extremely drunk and seemed totally confused."

When John saw his nurse and her husband standing there, he stopped and stared at them. After a moment, he slowly lowered the shotgun, staggered into the living room, and fell into a chair. Jay walked toward him very carefully while speaking calmly. He reached over and took the gun from John's lap. The physician lowered his head and just sat there.

At the same time, Dallas hurried upstairs and found Dot stuck in a bedroom window. When the terrified housewife saw her friend, she screamed, "Keep him away from me!"

"I was afraid she was going to fall out the window," the nurse recalled, "so I ran over and quickly pulled her back inside. We were in one of the boys' rooms. We sat on the edge of the bed and it took a little while before she stopped shaking. Then she began to cry. Finally I helped her lie down and she eventually went to sleep.

"My husband also got Dr. Mooney into bed downstairs. Jay and I spent the night dozing on the sofa. We wanted to make sure nothing was going to start up again. They were still both asleep when we left early in the morning."

That Monday at the office, the physician showed up on time for his appointments and never said a word about what had happened that weekend. Even later that day, when Dot called to make sure her husband made it to the office, nothing was said about the scary event. The nurse often wondered if both of them had been in blackouts and didn't remember a thing.

Those kinds of sudden and irrational outbursts continued to take their toll on all three of the Mooney youngsters.

"I think it might have had an effect on me emotionally," Al Mooney admits. "In fact, I know it did. I became what I call an emotional pack rat. Since I didn't have parents to bounce things off of, I stuffed a lot of my feelings. I believe I've been pretty sane and level-headed since I've grown up, but I know I have issues. I suspect they relate back to some of my upbringing as a child."

Being the oldest, Al says his parents' erratic behavior literally terrified him and his brothers at times, particularly some of the strange things his father was apt to do. One summer day, for example, John took his sons and a few of their friends to Savannah Beach. He drove with the top down on his white Thunderbird convertible knowing that his sons enjoyed it. He was making another attempt at being a good father.

He had some beers at the beach but didn't appear to be the least bit intoxicated as they headed for home. Still, his actions turned out to be somewhat questionable for a sober man.

Halfway back to Statesboro, it began to rain quite heavily. Instead of putting up the convertible top, the physician decided to give the boys "a real thrill." He accelerated his Thunderbird to over a hundred miles an hour so that the rain deflected off the windshield and blew over the car. Some of the youngsters were a bit white-faced by the time they got home.

Later, when Al mentioned what had happened to his mother—thinking he was heaping manly praise on his dad—Dot became very angry. She told her husband that he could have skidded in the rain, smashed into a tree, and killed everyone in the car. They argued for hours until John had had enough to drink and went to bed.

But Al likes to point out that there were some positive things about growing up in a dysfunctional family: "If you spend a lot of your time in your room trying to isolate from all the chaos around you like I did, there's plenty of time to read and study. In a way, that probably made me a pretty good student. I'd say that, to a degree, the isolation I experienced in my younger years impacted me in a positive way as an adult."

Today Dr. Al J. Mooney is recognized as one of the leading addiction specialists in the country in the book *The Best Doctors in America*. He has thirty years of experience in the treatment of alcoholism and drug addiction and is currently practicing addiction medicine in his private practice in Raleigh, North Carolina. He is also the coauthor of the best-selling treatise on addiction called *The Recovery Book*.

"As a kid, I really looked up to my brother Al," said Jimmy Mooney, the middle son. "It was like he always did everything right. He excelled in school and seemed to be the perfect son—always helping my parents whenever he could. So when he would get into trouble with them over nothing, I couldn't understand it. So I just kept quiet and kept my head down."

That's why Jimmy says he also isolated as a young boy: "I never wanted to rock the boat because you never knew what was going to happen if you rocked the boat. I just wanted everything at home to be nice and calm. I never wanted to upset my mother or father. I knew what it could lead to."

He also remembers being shielded from many of the family disruptions by his grandparents and also by "Aunt Honey" and "Uncle Bill." When trouble broke out, he would be scooped up along with his brothers and taken to more pleasant places until the storm subsided. Looking back at all that erratic behavior now, he said: "It seemed like most of the time I was an outsider looking in. I probably would have been more horrified and been more affected had I paid attention to all the arguments and all the fighting. I guess I was able to turn away from a lot of it, to pretend it wasn't really that bad. Strange as it may sound, being a kid growing up in that kind of atmosphere, it just seemed pretty normal to me most of the time."

Bobby Mooney, the youngest, was only about four or five years old when the worst of the nightmares occurred, so he remembers very little—only that he was well cared for by his parents and all those around him.

"While I can't really recall any of the grief they may have given me as a kid," he said, "I sure can remember the grief I gave them when I got a little older and got into alcohol and drugs myself. Maybe that's why they understood so well what I had to go through because they had gone through it themselves."

After recovering from the disease of alcoholism and drug abuse many years ago, Dr. Robert W. Mooney also decided to devote his life to addiction medicine and the treatment of alcoholics, drug addicts, and their family members affected by chemical dependence. He is a Diplomate of the American Board of Addiction Medicine and a Diplomate of the American Psychotherapy Association. He is both a licensed physician and a licensed psychiatrist.

John and Dot Mooney would be immensely proud today of all three of their sons and their dedication to stemming the tide of the disease that nearly ruined their lives. However, Dot in particular regretted for a long time what she had done because all she ever wanted to be was a good wife and a good mother.

Dallas Cason attested to Dot's desire without hesitation: "She really loved her children and despite her terrible addiction, she tried to be there for them most of the time when they were growing up."

In comparison, the trusted nurse was there for Dr. Mooney all the time. In fact, at one point, she found herself in serious trouble professionally for trying to do too much in order to preserve what was left of his medical practice. As she explained, "Most of Dr. Mooney's patients had been coming to see him for years. He even brought many of them into this world. They loved and respected him and he knew their medical needs. So when he started being away from the office for longer and longer periods of time, they would come and talk to me before going to see another doctor.

"I remember there was a music professor from a local college. He had a hearing problem because of the excess wax he had in his ears. He wouldn't let anyone irrigate his ears but Dr. Mooney or me. He used to say that we helped him to hear every single note in the music he was teaching. So even when Dr. Mooney was gone, he came to see me for his treatments.

"And then there was this retired navy doctor who would get vitamin B12 shots occasionally. So I continued giving them to him. If people needed injections that required a prescription, I would call Dr. Daniel and describe the shot Dr. Mooney usually gave the patient. He would tell me how to prescribe for it. I would do so and then give the injection to the patient."

While Dallas knew she was handling more and more of the medical procedures the missing physician would normally perform himself, she was so intent on holding things together that she didn't realize she might be exceeding her boundaries as a nurse—that is, until one afternoon when a Georgia state medical official showed up at the office. His name was Mr. Clifton and he was from the State of Georgia Medical Registration Board, the official body that issued licenses for doctors and nurses and anyone or anything related to the practice of medicine.

"He was there to pick up my nurse's license," Dallas said, still sounding a bit shocked by the recollection. "He had heard somehow about all I was doing in the absence of Dr. Mooney and said it was against the law. He explained that I was not supposed to prescribe anything for anybody or give certain kinds of shots or perform certain procedures without the doctor being present. I asked if I could speak with him for a moment and explain the situation I was in. He agreed to listen."

She said the state official turned out to be a very kind and understanding man. He had been with the state board for many years and knew that Dr. Mooney was a very well-respected physician among his peers. After the nurse explained that the physician was off getting help before his condition worsened, the official relented in his decision.

"He said it would be okay for me to keep doing what I was doing until the doctor returned," Dallas said. "He simply made me promise not to overstep my nursing responsibilities any further than I already had in treating patients. I assured him I wouldn't and he left without taking away my license."

Shortly after John returned from another sabbatical, the office was visited by not one threatening medical representative but by a whole group, much to the physician's chagrin. It was in the early spring of 1959, and as the hard-pressed doctor would tell the story about the incident sometime later, "The supply line for all the drugs I was using was beginning to close up. The scheme I had going with the six drugstores in Statesboro that had worked so well for a number of years was finally unraveling.

"I used to go from one drugstore to the next, ordering prescription medications that were allegedly for my patients but were actually for me. I thought that if I kept rotating my orders from one store to another, none of them would catch on. That's how smart I thought I was. Rather, it was how much my addiction was now affecting my brain.

"I was writing out phony prescriptions for Demerol and Dilaudid and other narcotics. I thought for a while that I was getting away with it even though I knew it was illegal. As time went by, I was sure that one day the feds would barge into my office, inspect my records, find most of them counterfeit, and haul me away in handcuffs. Little did I expect that it would be the local drugstore owners who would barge in first."

But that's what happened. Some of the owners had begun comparing notes. As a result, the alarm bells went off and all six of them showed up at the medical office in a bunch.

"You're ordering more narcotics from us than all of the other doctors in Statesboro combined," one of them said in a surprisingly friendly tone. "You're ordering almost as many as we send to the hospital. We don't know what you're doing with all these drugs, but you're going to have to get them somewhere else from now on because we are no longer supplying you."

Looking back at the incident some years later, the addicted physician came to realize that these druggists were doing one of the greatest things they could for him. They were pointing out the seriousness of his problem without even saying so directly. The message they gave him was to have a profound effect on him eventually.

"Here were six of my friends," John would say later, "that I always thought were loyal to me but now seemed to be turning against me. I was disappointed at first by their decision, but I knew they were right."

Still, that difficult confrontation with six meaningful friends didn't change a thing. It takes more than sincere caring and sensible words to eliminate the cravings of addiction. So it didn't take long before the ailing physician came up with yet another scheme.

He still had his state-approved narcotics stamp at his office. At that time, provided you had an approved stamp and properly filled-out requisition forms, you could order narcotics from drug wholesalers and they would ship them to you directly. All you had to do was make sure you kept records on each and every transaction.

John began ordering hundreds of pills at a time, writing fictitious names on the forms and keeping no records. He felt he didn't need to keep any records since he was the only one taking the drugs. However, forged names on counterfeit requisition forms and no records to boot violated both state and federal laws—and John knew it. That's why he started traveling to drug wholesale houses in other towns and cities so that he wouldn't be found out as he had been by the pharmacists in Statesboro.

Even though his scheme appeared to be working rather well, the jittery surgeon soon became very worried once again. Since he sometimes ordered a thousand pills at a time, he was afraid some wholesaler might get suspicious and begin checking into his own records. So he stopped doing business with the wholesalers and launched into what he called his "panhandling period."

"I started seeing a variety of doctors in other towns," he once explained. "I would make up symptoms and get them to write me prescriptions for some real heavy-duty narcotics. Then I'd go to drugstores in those towns to get them filled. It wasn't as difficult as I thought it might be and it was a whole lot safer. At least that's what I told myself."

One day John was in Savannah scouting out more doctors when he bumped into one of his former patients, a woman who had moved to Savannah a few years before. She said she had a good job at the Dream House Furniture Company on Bay Street. She invited him to visit the place if he was ever in the area so she could show him around. He said he would, but then dismissed the idea.

"The next day I was cruising through Savannah again, checking on the locations of a few doctors I planned to see," he went on. "I happened to pass by Bay Street and spotted the Dream House Company on the corner. Then I noticed there was a large drugstore right next to it. I thought to myself, I bet that woman knows that druggist."

So the great manipulator stopped and went into the furniture store. After his former patient gave him a brief tour, the physician mentioned that he was thirsty.

"Is there somewhere nearby where we might get a soda?" he asked, knowing full well what the answer would be.

"Right next door at the druggist," she replied.

As they drank their Cokes, Dr. Mooney told the woman that on his way back to Statesboro, he had to pay a visit to a young girl who had cancer.

"She'll be requiring some narcotics for her pain," he explained. "I'd like to purchase them here in Savannah, but I can't unless someone can identify me as a doctor. I mean, I have my business card, but since you were one of my patients . . ."

John didn't even have to finish his sentence before the woman gladly volunteered to tell the druggist that he was her former family doctor—"and a very good one at that," she added. She then took him to the counter and introduced him to a very nice young man.

After shaking hands, John repeated his story about his alleged cancer patient. The druggist said that ordinarily he would need to see some official identification. However, since his good customer could vouch that John was a doctor in good standing, there wouldn't be a problem.

"Tell me, Doctor," the young druggist said, "exactly what is it you need?"

John Mooney was surprised at how smoothly the transaction went. As he said later, "I simply pulled out my prescription pad and ordered a significant quantity of Demerol for a young girl who didn't exist. I even talked that druggist into letting me pay for the prescription myself, saying I would have the girl's family reimburse me later."

Once again the druggist agreed. In a very short time, the addicted physician walked out of that drugstore and headed for home with so much Demerol that he didn't have to see any more doctors for quite awhile—in Savannah or anywhere else.

For some reason, however, the transaction at that pharmacy in Savannah began to haunt John Mooney. He started to think about the six drugstore owners in Statesboro. He knew they suspected that many of the prescriptions he wrote were bogus. But they were his friends and he knew they didn't want to report him to the authorities. Writing prescriptions for a fictitious person makes one liable for up to five years in a federal prison and at least two years without parole in a Georgia state correctional facility. John was fully aware of this.

"I started waking up at night in a cold sweat," the anxious doctor often recalled. "Part of it was the drinking and the drugging, I know, but the other part was the horrible fears I had of being caught and sent to prison. And I knew that if I didn't get off this merry-go-round, that's exactly where I would end up."

John would get out of bed in the middle of the night, go into the kitchen, and pour himself a drink. Then he would begin chain-smoking as he paced up and down. He was obsessed by his fears. Everything was in shambles and he saw no way out. He had tried everything he knew to cure what he still believed was a mental condition and nothing had worked.

He would squeeze his fists against his temples, trying to squash out the images of his frightened children, his frantic wife, his bewildered nurse, and the stares of former friends that would fill him with shame. There was no order of any sort in his life. It was totally unmanageable. There was nothing left but confusion and chaos.

On one of those terrible nights when his drinking and drugging and smoking and pacing did not bring him the slightest semblance of sleep or a brief moment of calm or peace, one last flicker of hope arose.

He suddenly remembered that a few months ago, shortly after he had checked himself into the Central of Georgia Hospital in Savannah to detox one more time, his good friend Dr. Jack Averitt came by to visit. Jack held a doctorate degree and was the dean of graduate studies at Georgia Southern College, as well as a church deacon, Sunday school teacher, organist, choir director, and soloist at the Statesboro First Baptist Church.

The highly respected university professor always seemed to be there when a friend or neighbor was in trouble. In fact, he had been dropping by the Mooneys' house of late to chat with Dot and pray with her and the children for their father's well-being. He was not only one of John's loyal childhood friends but had been one of his very patient patients for a long, long time.

As the trembling physician sat there in the darkened kitchen, he clearly recalled the serious look on Jack's face that afternoon, a look he had never seen before. At first John tried to crack a few jokes, but the frown on the professor's brow only grew deeper. This time Jack wasn't buying his bedridden friend's lies about being in the hospital for a peptic ulcer. Instead, he got right to the point.

"It's not your stomach I'm concerned about, John," he said in a strong but obviously nervous tone. "I should have told you this a long time ago, but I can't ignore your problem anymore. I'm concerned about your alcoholism and drug addiction, and it's time you did something about it. I mean something serious about it."

It would have hurt less had this particular friend hit him over the head with a sledgehammer or spit in his face. John had always prided himself in having Dr. Jack Averitt's respect. It meant something to the way he felt about himself—being on a par with an intellectual who was highly regarded in the community. Now that was gone too. He could feel the anger and rage filling his gut and fogging his brain. It poured out in a string of profane and derogatory remarks he seemed to have no control over. It concluded with a demand that the professor "get the hell out of this goddam room right now and don't ever come back!"

Instead, his friend moved closer to his bed.

"No!" Jack said quite emphatically. "We've been friends for a long time and I deserve to be heard. So does Miss Dallas, that loyal nurse of yours you couldn't get along without. She told me about all these fancy country club places you've been landing in to dry out—and if you fire her for telling me, then you're not the man I think you are, John Mooney.

"All we want to do is help you. Dallas found a place where you might finally get rid of this curse that's killing you and wrecking your whole family."

While the seriously impaired physician grabbed the sides of his bed, trying to control his rage, Dr. Averitt went on to tell him about a special hospital for drug addiction in Lexington, Kentucky, that only handled the toughest cases.

"I hear it's a very difficult place to be," Jack concluded, "but maybe that's what you need. And I promise to stand by you all the way. So for God's sake, John, give it a try." Then he turned and walked out of the room.

John never said a word about Jack's visit to Dallas Cason upon his return to Statesboro. It was an event he intended to forget completely. When he started another bout with alcohol and drugs the next day, it helped him to do just that.

But now in his darkened kitchen, as he rose and began pacing again, he remembered not only his confrontation with his dear friend that day in Savannah but also a more recent visit from a new patient who had once been a morphine addict. The man had told him he had tried the cure in many places, but that nothing worked until he checked himself into the U.S. Public Health Services Hospital in Lexington, Kentucky—the very place Jack and Dallas had told him about. The morphine addict said the hospital first straightened out his thinking and then cured him of his addiction.

Before his patient left that day, John remembered him saying, "I've been clean now for over five years thanks to that place in Kentucky and I ain't ever going back to drugs ever again."

The physician stopped pacing, went upstairs, and woke his wife. When Dot saw the look on her husband's face, she thought at first that he was hallucinating again. When she discovered he wasn't, she began to listen to his story about the drug hospital in Lexington.

"I've been to all kinds of fancy places up and down the East Coast," he said to his wife with tears streaming down his face.

"I've spent lots of money and it has gotten me nowhere. I remember Jack Averitt and this other patient of mine saying it was a real tough place but that people had gotten better there and stayed better. I believe it now, Dot, and I'm at the end of my ropes. That's why I'm going."

Dot pulled her husband close to her and they cried each other to sleep.

Two days later, on Friday, June 15, 1959, Dr. John Mooney Jr. was on his way to Lexington, Kentucky.

CHAPTER NINE

There's No Way Out

HE COULD HAVE FLOWN TO LEXINGTON, KENTUCKY, OR TAKEN a train or a bus. Or he could have called Dr. Jack Averitt to drive him there. He was sure Jack would have done it. But John was still embarrassed by their last encounter in Savannah. He promised himself he would apologize to his friend upon his return. So, the rather depressed and somewhat unsteady physician decided to take the almost six-hundred-mile trip by himself in his 1956 white Ford Thunderbird with its red convertible top.

John Mooney needed something to keep him focused that day, something that could prop up his spirits and make him feel good about himself and what he was about to do. He needed to feel that all hope was not lost, and that maybe, just maybe, he would find the real answer to his problems in what he envisioned would be a cold and rugged asylum designed to cure the worst addicts on the planet.

Yes, he needed to feel better about himself, and he hadn't done so in a very long time.

But there had always been one exception, at least since 1956—his

Ford T-Bird. Flying across the country in his white Thunderbird always made him feel a little bit better. That's why he decided to drive it to Lexington. Although he was reluctant to admit it to himself, this sleek white Thunderbird represented his last vestige of success, his "cover," if you will, for his abject failure as a husband, a father, and a physician. It was his outer garment that shouted "You're still somebody" over the purring sound of its V-8 engine: "I'm still Dr. John Mooney, Jr. I'm still a skilled surgeon and good doctor who owns a Ford Thunderbird. Yes, I've made a few mistakes along the way. But now I plan to fix those mistakes, get back on the right track, and stay there."

As he pressed down on the gas pedal and watched the pointer on the 150-mph speedometer climb easily past 60, he felt his confidence rise along with it. The T-Bird was doing its job. Strange as it may seem, that's exactly what this 1956 Ford Thunderbird was created to do according to its designers—to make the owner feel special in this uniquely crafted automobile.

Yes, it was a special car for special people that hit the market at a time when John Mooney needed a big change in his life. It was only a few years earlier that the American auto industry was in the doldrums. For a man like John who loved cars, there was nothing around that stood out from the pack. A car was a car was a car. A Ford was a Ford. A Chevrolet was a Chevrolet. They made sedans, coupes, station wagons, and convertibles. All were simply straightforward variations of a common design. A dilettante might say they were boring machines that drove you further into boredom.

Then in 1955, the Ford Thunderbird exploded onto the scene. It ignited the first real excitement in the American auto industry since Henry Ford introduced the Model-T. It delivered the kind of style and sophistication that used to be available only in expensive imports like the Mercedes-Benz and the Jaguar, and it did it at a reasonable price tag compared to its European counterparts.

Evoking the mythological creature of America's indigenous

people, the Thunderbird was a sporty, two-seat convertible with a starting price of $2,695 that could run up to $3,800 with options. Ford called it "the personal car" when it was first introduced at the Detroit Auto Show in February 1954. When it finally came rolling off the assembly line in October of that year as a 1955 model, it created a brand-new market for such cars and a sales boom far beyond the company's forecast.

By the time word got to Statesboro, Georgia, about this unique and classy new car, sales had depleted all available 1955 models. So John quickly put in his order for a 1956 white Thunderbird with a red convertible top. He wanted the classiest and most prestigious model available.

As the Ford Motor Company had done the year before with the introduction of their sensational new vehicle, buyers were once again invited to Detroit to watch their own T-Birds roll off the assembly line and to select whatever special options they desired. John quickly accepted the invitation. He flew up to Detroit and was there at the assembly plant to watch the last piece of trim firmly affixed to his new pride and joy.

He signed the ownership papers, received the keys, climbed into the sporty vehicle, and proudly drove home to Statesboro.

It wasn't that the troubled physician needed this sleek, athletic-looking white T-Bird to show off to his friends and neighbors. He already knew they respected him for his medical skills and attention to their needs. He even knew they forgave him for his lapses. John needed this special car for himself, to make himself feel special, to help salve those deep-seated feelings of low self-esteem he still felt at times.

That's why the physician decided to drive to Lexington that day in his "personal car." Even though it was now almost three years old and had a few what you might call "drinking dents" in its bumpers, this white T-Bird was still doing the job it was designed to do for people like John Mooney.

What also helped build his spirits as he headed north through the Smoky Mountains of Tennessee into the bluegrass horse country of Kentucky was the bright sunshine that filled a cloudless blue sky. It was a spectacular spring day that filled him with hope and anticipation.

"I looked sort of gray from all the stuff I had been taking," he once said about his trip, "so I had the convertible top down to get a little suntan. I wanted to get some color in my face so that when I arrived they didn't think I was a corpse and bury me alive."

The clean fresh air blowing across John's face also awakened his memory to some things he had forgotten about his conversation with the morphine addict that day in his office. He suddenly remembered the man saying the U.S. Public Health Service Hospital he went to in Lexington was a small part of a big complex that included a large drug prison right next to it. People were incarcerated there for serious drug felony offenses.

John's foot slowly eased back off the gas pedal as he took a moment to digest this newly remembered information. So what's the problem? he reasoned. He was going there of his own volition, volunteering to be treated for his addiction. He wasn't charged with any criminal offenses—at least not yet—so he should expect to be treated just as his morphine-addicted friend was and hopefully leave the place with the same outcome. Some years later, the physician remembered hearing a little voice in his head at that moment reminding him of something else.

You've been spending a whole lot of money on places you can't afford and what was the result? You're in worse shape than ever. This place will be free. You've been going to expensive places where they dress for dinner, where they wear tuxedos and evening dresses, and where they carve the meat for you at dinner. You've been associating with a group of emotionally ill people that your pride keeps telling you they're your type. They're presidents of insurance companies and banks and big corporations and you're a big-shot doctor, or so you think. No, John, you need to be with really sick people like the kind I'm sure you'll find in Lexington.

So he decided to continue on. As he pushed back down on the gas pedal, he knew how much trouble could lie ahead if he didn't give this hospital an honest try. He promised himself he would enter as a volunteer and stay until he was cured of his habit. Okay, maybe he really didn't want to stop drinking forever, but he sure as heck did want to quit the drugs. They were killing him. He was sick and tired of how they controlled his life.

"I knew in my heart I was deadly earnest about this," the physician once said. "So I think this was the point where God decided he might be able to help me. When I look back now, I can see it was a beginning. But I'm mighty grateful that God is patient, for it took me awhile from that point to finally get well."

What John didn't realize at the time was that God wasn't the only one trying to help him. So were many of his friends and fellow workers back in Statesboro.

His nurse, Dallas Cason, for example, was still trying to keep his medical practice going by treating whatever patients she could on her own. When their problems appeared to be more serious than she could handle, she would suggest they see John's good friend Dr. Bird Daniel until Dr. Mooney returned.

His attorney, George Johnston, was fending off the physician's creditors as best he could, including the Internal Revenue Service.

And then of course there was Dr. Jack Averitt, who was delighted when Dot called him to say that her husband was finally admitting himself into a facility that might be able to help him. In fact, Jack dropped by to see Dot that afternoon and tell her how pleased he was. His warmth and comfort left her with a feeling that, if things should ever get a whole lot worse, this was one person she could truly count on.

It was dusk when John finally arrived outside the ominous-looking gray walls of what the locals in the area called the "Narcotics Farm," which encompassed both the hospital and the notorious federal prison for drug offenders. John later explained the outcome of his experience at the public health hospital this way: "I expected to be admitted as Dr. John Mooney Jr., the distinguished surgeon from south Georgia. But it didn't happen just like that."

The guard at the gate asked, "What's your term up here for?"

John replied: "Well, I thought I'd come up here for a little while on a voluntary basis and get some treatment."

"Treatment for what?"

"Well, I have a nervous disorder. It's a constant nervous condition and I take some medication for it. But I haven't taken any in a long time."

The guard pointed to the passenger side of the white T-Bird and asked, "What's that stuff on the front seat of your car?"

John looked down and saw a whole bunch of pills all over the front seat and on the floor of his car. He hadn't even noticed they were there during his entire trip to Kentucky. He looked back up rather sheepishly to see the guard smirking. "Go right up that driveway," he said, "and they'll take you in."

"So I followed his directions," John continued, "and drove up this small hill to a tall brick building with ivy growing all over it. Two men in white uniforms met me at the front door to the hospital. One of them took my bags while the other one helped me out of the car, then got in and drove it off, I guess to park it somewhere. I crossed my fingers they wouldn't damage it.

"Inside, the man put a big metal band around my suitcases, locked the band and stamped it. He told me they were being put into storage and would be safe until I was ready to leave. When I said I needed some things from my bags, the man shook his head, then led me to a room where a nurse handed me some underwear and two white uniforms, the same kind I noticed patients in the nearby hallway were wearing.

"Then they had me sign my name in a big book and told me to take off all my clothes and put on one of the white uniforms. I was humiliated. I was mortified. I tried to tell them I was a doctor with an above average education and held three college degrees.

That I was a fellow of the American College of Surgeons and had medical papers published. But it didn't seem to make any difference. No one was listening.

"Finally, dressed in this wrinkled white uniform that was much too tight for me, they led me down a rather musty hallway toward my room. As I looked around, it finally struck me that I was now in a place with people who were really like myself— people who just weren't acquainted with reality, who lived like I did much of the time in some fantasy world someplace far away. I was in drug land, U.S.A.

"I hardly had time to go to the bathroom before the man who had taken my bags came into my room and accompanied me to a large dining area filled with patients gobbling down food from steel trays. I hadn't eaten all day, so I filled my tray and found a seat next to a rather large man with heavy black stubble all over his face. He was wearing a different colored uniform. It was gray and had black numbers printed across the front and back. I noticed some others dressed the same way. I found out later they were from the prison unit and came to the hospital to be treated for their drug problems.

"As I reached across the table to pick up the saltshaker, the rather large man bounced back in his chair and raised his fist toward me. I thought he was going to kill me right then and there. Instead he glared at me and said in a menacing voice, 'We're polite around here. We try to be courteous. That saltshaker was sitting right in front of my plate. You should have asked me to pass it. Don't you never as long as you live insult me that way again.'

"I looked up at him and gulped. I promised I would never do that again. Then I looked back down at my tray. I had quickly lost my appetite. So I excused myself and went back to my room. On the way out I could hear some men laughing at me and realized the rather large gent was only messing with me. But it made me begin to question whether or not I really wanted to be in a place like this. It might not cost anything, but there could be another kind of price to pay. By the time I got back to my room, I was already thinking of ways to get out of there.

"I started hearing that voice in my head again and it was telling me these really weren't my kind of people at all. These people have no compassion for what I'm going through. Why on earth would they put a distinguished physician like me in the same room with a bunch of dope fiends from the prison? And I'll be with them in the same treatment sessions. It's humiliating. I just can't do it."

But John had told Dot that morning as he left that he would stay in this place for a year if necessary, regardless of what it was like, just as long as it was helping him get better. What would he say to her now after being there less than a day? She was already at her wit's end with him and having difficulty with her own problems. So he took a deep breath and decided he could hang in there for a week or so. He would consider that to be an honest effort on his part. And if he decided to leave, then hopefully Dot would understand.

John actually gave it ten days before he threw in the towel. It took that long to physically withdraw from the effects of all the drugs in his system.

When you refuse to approach a difficult treatment program with an open mind, ten days can seem like a thousand years. And that's how it was for a physician who kept tripping over his ego and pride everywhere he went. His appointed psychiatrist tried everything from kindness to understanding and from insults to threats but soon realized he was working on a hopeless case. He was dealing with a patient who had all the answers but didn't understand any of the questions. So on June 29, 1959, the doctor sat down with John for a brief but decisive talk. His now angry and disillusioned patient wasted no time expressing his feelings.

"Your so-called recovery program here is nothing but a form of shock treatment," he said. "It may work on people like my wife, but it's certainly not going to work on me. I can't identify with anybody around this place. I've treated dope fiends myself as a doctor, but some of these guys go way beyond being dope fiends. I want out of here now!"

His doctor calmly replied: "You came here voluntarily, Dr. Mooney, so you are free to leave at any time. However, if you decide to leave, you are going to leave AMA. That means 'against medical advice.' You'll have to sign a paper saying that's why you're leaving.

"And I'll tell you furthermore that if you don't stay now, when there's no pressure on you from any legal authorities, I predict you'll be back here inside of a year with drug felony charges hanging all over you. So if you think it's been difficult for you so far, you haven't seen anything if you decide to leave."

Four little words kept running through John's mind as he sat there listening to his counselor: "This guy's a nut." When the man was finished, the angry physician signed the AMA paper, gathered up his belongings, and left. Later in life he described that episode in Lexington this way:

"I left that place determined I would never take another drug. For some reason, I really did feel a release from my obsession. When you finally leave a place like that, I guess it's only natural to feel good just to be free. My pride had been bruised, but once I put on my suit, my shirt, and my tie—what I called my executive look—I wiped it away by simply admitting I had made another dumb mistake.

"And so I got into my white T-Bird and drove back down route US 25, thinking how great it was not ever having to go back in there. All I had to do was stay off alcohol and drugs and I wouldn't have to wind up in any more treatment places, especially one like that. For a man like me, with my willpower, my education, with my mind, it shouldn't be all that difficult. I just hadn't been putting enough effort into it. I should thank God I went there because I now saw what could happen should I ever have another relapse.

"So I promised myself one more time that I would never again

as long as I lived ever touch a drink of liquor or ever take a narcotic shot or a tranquilizer pill or a sedative anymore, under any
circumstances. And as soon as I made that promise, my pride that
had been bruised in that awful hospital was immediately soothed
and I felt once again that I now had complete control over my life.

"As I continued down Route 25, I enjoyed watching the trees
whizzing by, listening to the birds chirping away, and seeing the
stately thoroughbred horses prancing across the thick Kentucky
bluegrass. It was beautiful. Then, rounding a curve, I spotted a
sign that read: LAST CHANCE TO BUY WHISKEY BEFORE KNOX-
VILLE, TENNESSEE.

"I saw the sign and smiled. For a moment it made no impression. Then my foot seemed to come off the gas pedal almost au-
tomatically as my sick brain went into action. I started thinking
about where was I headed and what was I going to do when I got
there.

"'John,' I told myself, 'it's getting late and you're going to have
to spend the night somewhere. And there's an old friend of yours
named Jim who lives in Gatlinburg, Tennessee, only about a hundred miles from here. He always said he would love to have you
come by if you were ever in the area.'

"'He was a real good friend in Statesboro before he moved to
Tennessee. I know he'd love to see you and he'd certainly put you
up for the night. But Jim likes to drink. It would only be hospi-
table of you to bring him a bottle of whiskey.'"

So the physician, who by now was a perfectionist in the art of
self-deception, turned off the road and found his way to the "Last
Chance" liquor store. He bought two fifths of Canadian Club and
put them next to him in the passenger seat. He felt good about
doing this favor for an old friend because he knew he wasn't going
to drink. He was just going to watch Jim enjoy the whiskey while
they talked about old times.

"Because I'm going to quit drinking doesn't mean everybody
else has to," he said to himself. "I'm not going to be a damper on

anyone's party. I want the people to carry on just like I was doing. If Jim likes a good drink, that's great. If Dot wants to drink now and then, let her. I'm not going to force my will on anybody else."

The conflicted physician was about ten miles or so back down the road when it occurred to him that Jim had sent him a letter a few months before saying he had moved from Gatlinburg, Tennessee, to Greenwood, South Carolina, about two years earlier. He had forgotten that letter. So here he was now stuck with all this liquor. It was too late to turn back to the store. He was already too many miles away.

So he decided to take it home and give it to Dot. He was still convinced she didn't have a serious problem with booze, only drugs. And besides, if she didn't want the liquor, she could always give it to one of her friends.

At Knoxville, Tennessee, John stopped at a hamburger joint to get something to eat. He left the top down on his T-Bird and took the whiskey in with him. He sat at a small table and ordered a hamburger and a Coca-Cola. His addicted mind started going again.

"'John,'" he thought, "'this is a wonderful thing you're doing, to realize you've thrown away half your life, probably more, and now you're going back home tomorrow to start staying sober for the rest of your life. That is truly a great, great thing. You ought to be proud of yourself.'"

The waitress brought over his hamburger and Coca-Cola. As he stared at the soda, his mind suddenly took another tack.

"'You know, John,'" he said to himself, "'if you're going to practice a lifetime of sobriety starting tomorrow, surely it won't hurt if you take one last little drink today.'"

He took the Coke and drank about half. Then he slowly glanced around the almost empty hamburger joint. No one was watching him. So he quietly removed a bottle of Canadian Club from the brown paper bag, uncorked the top, and poured it into the soda until the glass was full.

"I started to drink it," he later recalled, "then I stopped. There was a moment of hesitation, but it wasn't strong enough to stop the process when you've become powerless over alcohol. So I drank it."

John didn't bother finishing his hamburger. He got up, put the liquor under his arm, threw a few bucks on the counter, and left. He knew he wasn't too many miles from Gatlinburg so he decided to spend the night at a motel there. He drove as fast as he could, trying hard not to think about what had just happened. But his conscience wouldn't let him. That voice in his head was back again.

"'John,'" the voice said, "'do you realize that a short time ago you made a decision to do something about your problem, and just a few hours ago you said you would never drink again as long as you live. And you've just taken a drink. What are you going to do now?'"

Surrender to the disease of addiction comes easily once you've taken the first drink or the first drug. As they say in Alcoholics Anonymous, one drink is too many and a thousand aren't enough. And that's the way it was with Dr. John Mooney as he sped toward Gatlinburg that afternoon. He knew in his mind, heart, and soul that he could no longer quit drinking or drugging. Had he been able to do it, he certainly would have done it under the terrible conditions at that hospital in Lexington.

"As an addict, there comes a time in your life, as it did in mine," the physician later explained, "when you use up all the willpower you have, all the strength and determination in your life in trying to do something, and then fail. So when I took that drink in that hamburger joint, I knew what had happened. I had lost the ability to control my own life. Panic set in because I knew somewhere deep inside I was headed for the worst drunk in my life and there was nothing, absolutely nothing I could do about it."

John not only got drunk that night in Gatlinburg, he woke

up the next morning in jail with what he called "striped sunshine coming through my window." He was charged with illegal parking for leaving his car halfway out in the road and also for public intoxication. He had enough money to pay the fine and started once again for home. But he was shaking so badly that he had to stop and buy more whiskey.

He got arrested again outside Columbia, South Carolina, where he spent two nights in jail, again for public drunkenness. A kind old country judge, learning the unshaven man before him was a doctor, let him off with a severe tongue-lashing. By the time John finally got back to Statesboro that evening, he was again very drunk and very angry—angry mostly at himself for having lost every bit of his pride, dignity and self-respect.

He was out of liquor and craving a drink. He staggered into his Lee Street house and started slamming open every kitchen cabinet in search of a bottle. He found a half-empty bottle of vodka under the sink. As he put it to his lips, he remembered seeing his now ten-year-old son, Al, standing in the doorway looking very sad. He heard him say, "Daddy, you're drunk again."

Then the boy turned and went back upstairs. John recalled taking a few more swigs from the bottle and then roaming around the house trying to find his wife. For some reason he began to sense that she had gone over to Honey and Bill Bowen's house, or maybe it was his son who told him that. He had expected her to be at home, to express some concern for his whereabouts and what had happened at the hospital. He concluded in his drunkenness that she just didn't give a damn.

So he was even angrier as he headed for the Bowens, bottle in hand. When he barged into their home, Bill, who was still the mayor of Statesboro, noticed that his usually amiable friend and neighbor was seething with rage. Honey saw a look on John's face she had never seen before. It frightened her. She became immediately concerned, not just for her husband and herself but for Dot as well. So she eased her way into the hall and called her friend Sheriff Harold Howell, who she knew would understand the situation they were in. She also quickly phoned Dr. Averitt, knowing of his close friendship with John and Dot.

"I had known Dr. Mooney practically all my life," the strong, stocky sheriff said, recalling that rather intense night. "He was somewhat older than me and had treated me several times in his office. I really respected him as a doctor.

"Later on, however, when his drinking and drugging got worse and I was called to his home at times to calm matters between him and Mrs. Mooney, our relationship became a bit strained. But I still respected him and wished I could do something to help him. So that night when Mrs. Bowen called and told me what was going on, I jumped into my car and got there as quickly as I could."

In the meanwhile, John had gotten into a fierce argument with Dot, who kept screaming at him, "I can't live with you anymore. You're driving me crazy." Every time Bill Bowen would try to intercede, the drunken physician would shove him aside and continue yelling at and threatening his wife.

"It was about nine o'clock at night when I got there," the sheriff remembered. "Dr. Averitt arrived just before me. I could hear John shouting all the way out into the street. I thought for a moment about getting some backup, but decided a big scene would only embarrass everyone. Besides, I felt I could probably calm him down since I had done it a few times before.

"When I entered the house, I could see the doctor was loaded to the gills and that he and the mayor were going at it back and forth. John was yelling at his wife, Dot, while Mr. Bowen and the professor were trying to console him and having very little luck. The mayor saw me and gave me a nod to take over. So I stepped in between them, looked John square in the face, and said to him, 'John, either you've got to calm down and come to your senses or I'm going to have to carry you out of here, put you in my car, and take you to jail.'

"I knew before the words were out of my mouth that it was a bad move. The doctor looked at me and growled, 'Not on your life!' Then he started rambling on about his wife not being home to take care of the kids and the Bowens always trying to interfere with his family. I kept trying to talk to him but he wouldn't listen. Then he and Dot got into another screaming match and I said to myself, that's it."

Sheriff Howell went back out to his radio car and called for his deputy, who arrived a few minutes later. They went back into the house together.

"I told the doctor he was coming with me," the sheriff continued. "He shoved me away and said if I was taking him to jail, he was going to call his lawyer, George Johnston, first. I said he could call him from my office. But John wouldn't give in. He staggered over to the telephone and picked up the receiver to dial. I followed him and pushed the button back down. He flew into a rage. He picked up the phone and threw it at me. If I hadn't ducked, he would have knocked my brains out with that phone. That was the last straw."

Sheriff Howell and his deputy grabbed John by the arms and dragged him outside to the front lawn, where they threw him down on the grass, accidentally breaking his eyeglasses. It was like a wrestling match until they finally got him into a straitjacket. Neighbors blocks away could hear the angry yells and curses coming from the mouth of a now helpless and drunken Dr. John Mooney Jr. It was a sad and sorry sight for so many people who cared deeply about this drowning man. Jack Averitt put it this way: "There are few situations that I have witnessed that were as tragic as the incident that took place that evening."

The sheriff finally managed to get John into his car and drove him off to jail. As he glanced back, he could see Dot Mooney standing at the front door of the Bowens' house, watching his car disappear down the street. Tears were streaming down her cheeks and there was pain and confusion etched across her face.

Everything within her sensed that all hope was gone. For despite this night and too many others like it, she still loved her husband, only now she felt exactly the same way he did—that there was truly no way out.

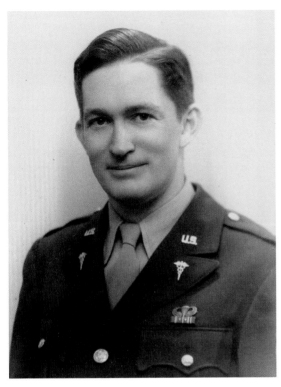

Captain John Mooney Jr., M.D.

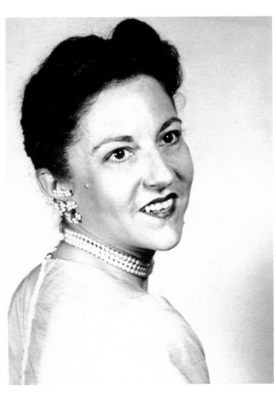

Dorothy Carolyn Riggs

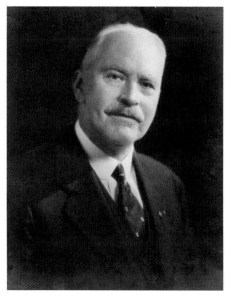

John's father.

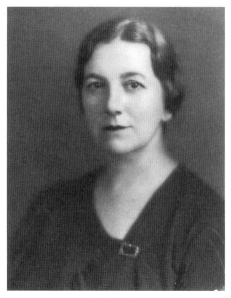

John's mother.

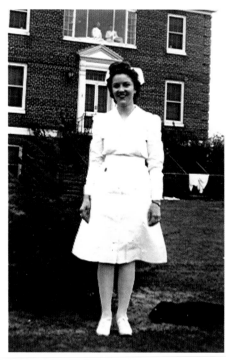

Dot as a nurse.

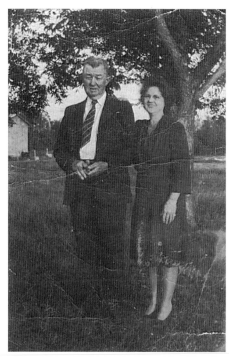

Dot's parents.

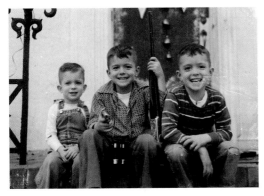

L-R: Bobby, Jimmy and Al.

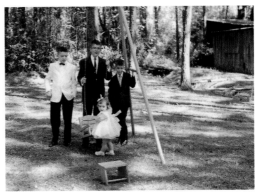

Swinging their baby sister, Carol Lind.

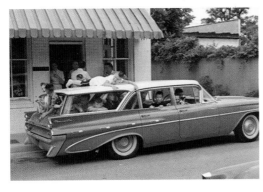

Preparing for a campout with her boys and their friends in Dot's station wagon.

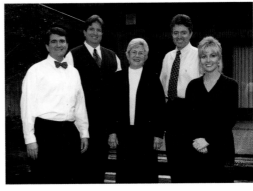

L-R: Dr. Al, Dr. Bobby, Dot, Jimmy, and Carol Lind Mooney.

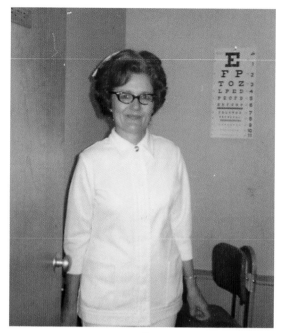

Nurse Dallas Cason

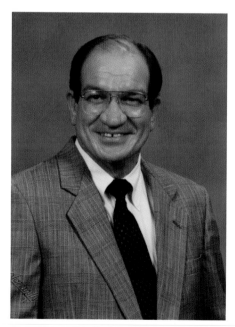

Earl Dabbs

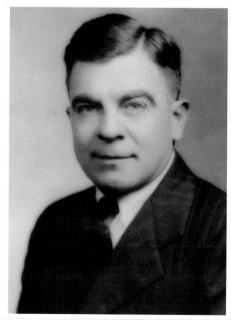

Houston Sewell

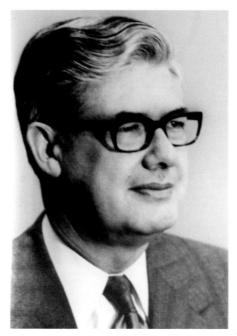

Dr. Jack Averitt

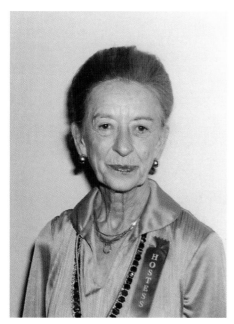

Honey Bowen

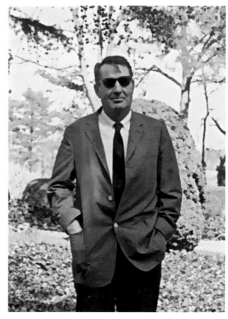

Bill Bowen

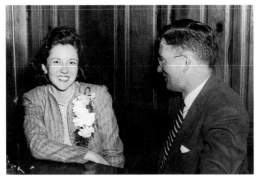

John and Dot shortly before their wedding.

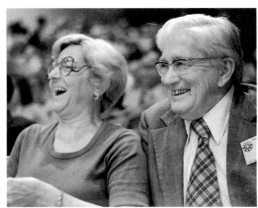

John and Dot enjoying sober years.

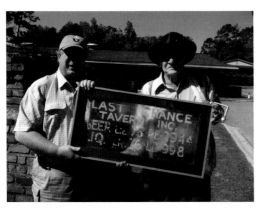

L-R: Dr. Bobby and friend David Odor hold replica of the "Last Chance Tavern" sign.

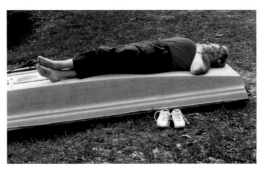

Dot at peace with her life.

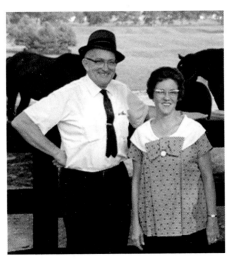

This picture was taken while John and Dot were visiting John's sponsor, Houston Sewell, in Lexington, Kentucky, and seeing the narcotics prison from which he had been released only fifteen months earlier.

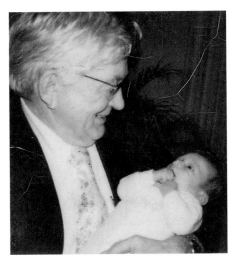

Dr. John holding his first grandchild, Alfonso John Mooney III.

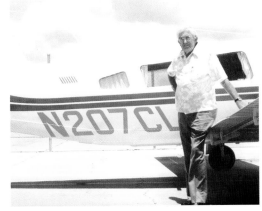

Dr. John loved to fly. Here he is posing with his airplane.

Dot Mooney helped many alcoholics find recovery, including this man who was so shaky at the time that she had to help him hold his glass to drink.

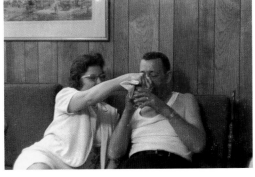
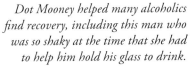

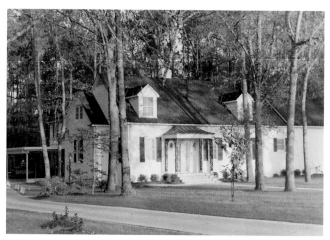

The "crazy" house on Lee Street where many alcoholics were saved.

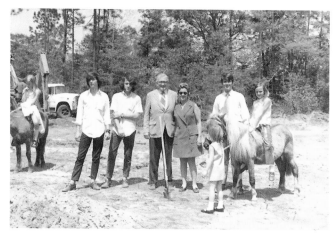

The Mooney family at informal groundbreaking ceremonies for Willingway.

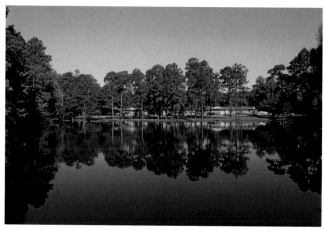

Willingway Hospital today.

CHAPTER TEN

A Man Worth Saving

JOHN MOONEY HAD COME TO IN A NUMBER OF JAIL CELLS BE-
fore, but awakening in the early morning hours of June 23, 1959,
in the Bulloch County Jail was an entirely different and somewhat horrific experience.

Both arms were partially numb and filled with pins and needles
from being harnessed in a straitjacket for so many hours. While
free from the painful device used primarily for the mentally ill—
which he felt added proof to his self-diagnosis as a nut case—he
lay there on the cold cement floor sweating and shaking. His throat
was parched and his mouth was caked with fragments of terrible-
tasting vomit. There was a noisy whirlwind in his head that finally lessened just a bit as he slowly pushed himself erect. But he
couldn't stop trembling.

Once again that morbid sense of doom surrounded him—that
overwhelming feeling of hopelessness and despair. Only this time
it was worse than he had ever experienced.

Many recovered alcoholics and drug abusers will tell you that
when someone suffering from the disease of addiction reaches this

state, which is often referred to as "the bottom," they are actually closer than they realize to exiting the hell they are in. Given the opportunity, they are ready to surrender to the truth. This once-respected physician, who now looked more like a Bowery derelict, was to be no exception.

For every drunk and drug addict, the turning point is different, yet it is the same. Crawling out of a deep, dark, dank pit of his or her own making is not an easy task. It requires help, like some force extending a loving hand, often through another person. But one has to reach out and grab hold.

In John Mooney's case, it was to be his estranged friend Dr. Jack Averitt who was to offer a loving hand. The sick and helpless physician was soon to discover that real friends don't just talk the talk—they actually walk the walk.

That terrible night before, when John was shamefully hauled off to jail kicking and screaming, those around him finally gave up, including his own wife. They felt there was no longer any way of saving someone who apparently didn't want to be saved. So again, they gave up.

But not Dr. Jack Averitt. As he stood on the sidewalk watching the sheriff's car drive off, he still believed in his heart that Dr. John Mooney Jr. was a man worth saving. So he said a prayer and then made himself a solemn promise—that he would go to any length to rescue this brilliant and talented surgeon who he knew was also a good and decent human being. How did he know that? Because that's what Jack Averitt was.

The next thing the university professor did that evening was to head across town to seek the support of John's minister, the Reverend Lawrence Houston, pastor of the Pittman Park Methodist Church. Despite the late hour, the clergyman invited Jack in but then seemed quite reluctant to discuss the current predicament of one of his parishioners. And when he finally did comment, Jack couldn't believe the words he heard coming from the minister's mouth: "I have spent so much time with John Mooney," he offered, "that I have neglected some of my other parishioners. I am sure that there is nothing that can be done to assist him. I consider Dr. Mooney to be a lost soul, and I cannot afford to spend any more time with him."

Totally bewildered by the attitude of this man of the cloth, Jack had to take a moment upon leaving to decide who to seek help from next. Since he knew his friend was very sick physically, as well as in mental and spiritual turmoil, he decided to call on Dr. Bird Daniel, who he knew was one of John's closest medical colleagues.

Dr. Daniel answered the door in his bathrobe. Jack was slightly embarrassed for calling on him so late in the evening; he apologized and asked if he could come back in the morning. When the doctor learned Jack was seeking his help for their mutual friend, their conversation turned out to be brief and to the point.

"You know, I've always admired and respected John's abilities," Dr. Daniel said in a sincere but very sad tone, "but we've all seen what his drinking and drugging have done to him. We have covered for him in the hospital all we are going to. He needs outside professional help. But the possibility of a doctor who is on alcohol and drugs withdrawing from the substance and maintaining a normal existence without it is highly improbable. I'm sorry, Dr. Averitt, but I think you have a lost cause on your hands."

It was after 11 p.m. by the time Jack returned home. His wife, Addie, was waiting up for him, anxious to hear what happened to Dr. Mooney. She had once been one of John's great admirers but had lost considerable respect for him over the past few years.

After her husband confided in her, she begged him not to get too deeply involved in "other people's messes." At the same time, she knew the man she married could never stand by and watch someone suffer if he could help in any way.

Shortly before 7 a.m., Dot called Jack. Her speech was a bit slurred as she explained she hadn't slept all night. She and John's younger sister, Sarah, who cared for him a great deal, had just returned from the Bulloch County Jail, where they found the physician so ill they were afraid he might die. Dot called Dr. Van Buren at Emory Medical Center in Atlanta; he had once been one of John's instructors at medical school and another great admirer of his talents. He suggested they send him immediately by ambulance to Grady Hospital in Atlanta, where he would look after him.

Jack quickly volunteered to go to Atlanta himself to see what else might be needed to help his friend recover—that perhaps just seeing a friendly face might buoy his spirits. He asked that Dot write a brief letter authorizing him to visit her husband just in case he ran into any red tape. Dot said she was so exhausted that no one would be able to read her hen scratching. She said she would call Dallas and ask her to write the letter and he could pick it up at John's office.

Feeling he had no time to waste, the professor managed to get a substitute to handle his classes that day, pick up the letter from Dallas, and still catch the 8:30 a.m. Nancy Hanks passenger train for the four-hour trip to Atlanta. He arranged to take the 6 p.m. train back and be home by 10:20 that same evening.

Once he boarded the train, relaxed in his seat, and started watching the familiar countryside roll by, Dr. Jack Averitt began asking himself what he would say to John Mooney this time. After all, what did he really know about the tragic malady that displayed itself so shockingly at the Bowens' house the night before? And how could he possibly influence in a positive way a man whose pastor and medical colleagues had already given up on, together with many in his own family? Was this purely an ego trip on his part, or did he feel honestly compelled by his God and his own nature to try at least to reach into the core of this once vital physician and touch his soul?

He thought about their relationship, how it began and what it had come to mean—thoughts he would expand upon in his journal once this emotional storm had passed:

"If one sets out to help another," he later wrote, "he must constantly evaluate whether it is for that person's benefit or for his own. What are his real motives? If he believes them to be truly unselfish, then he is compelled to proceed.

"Alfonso John Mooney Jr. was a neighbor of mine growing up. He was a bit older but we became good friends. I developed a sincere appreciation and admiration for his talents. The Mooney family lived on the northwest corner of North Main and Olliff streets in a very handsome house. John was reared with everything that one could desire, an environment complementary to his native ability and multiplicity of talents.

"He was described by young and old alike as brilliant and the prognosis for his success was positive in every respect. He became something of a hero of mine because his associates and friends recognized his outstanding qualities and I enjoyed being in his company.

"After completing Statesboro High School with an exceptional record, John went to Emory Medical School and became an outstanding physician and an exceptional surgeon. His life seemed to be ordered to the highest plateau of success. He even married well, to an Atlanta debutante who was the great-granddaughter of Joseph E. Brown, the Governor of Georgia during the Civil War.

"His choice was to return to Statesboro to open his medical practice here even though his professors at Emory predicted he could have a great practice in one of the state's larger cities. But he decided to return home and his scintillating and persuasive personality, together with his genuine interest and concern for his patients, made him an immediate success.

"On one occasion when a young man was involved in an accident and required extensive surgery, I heard one of Statesboro's citizens remark, 'I hope the family chose John Mooney for the surgery. He's the best in the whole southeast.'

"On the surface, John's personal life seemed to complement his professional career. He and his wife, Sally, built a lovely home on Lee Street. The town conversation reported that each room was built to accommodate the antique furnishings that Sally inherited from her family. When completed, it was a little gem.

"John and I were in the Statesboro Music Club together. He was a wonderful violinist and I was an adequate soloist. Our close association gave my wife Addie and I the opportunity to visit John and Sally's home on numerous occasions. Had I been assigned the task to name the ideal couple and the unsurpassed environment in which they lived and worked, I would have selected John and Sally Mooney.

"And then the war came. John quickly signed up and was highly qualified to meet the rigorous requirements of the medical corps to which he was assigned. He became a paratrooper and was often dropped ahead of the battle lines to care for the thousands of wounded soldiers. There was no doubt that this was a strenuous, tense and frustrating period in the life of one whose capabilities were equal to the task. My admiration for him grew enormously.

"And then the war was over and John Mooney came home a different man. The whole town praised him as the hero he was, but also quietly discussed the effects the war had on him. It was almost unanimously agreed that parachuting behind the lines, taking care of the wounded and dying and getting wounded twice yourself was a reasonable explanation for the change in his behavior.

"Then rumors began about John and Sally. She had suddenly moved back to her parents' home in Atlanta without any explanation. Since rumors at first are simply myths in quest of reality, the reality finally came in the legal actions filed with the Clerk of the Court of Bulloch County—a divorce action between John and Sally. Some folks were shocked. Others who knew more weren't.

"However, there was no hiding the fact that whatever the cause of their breakup, it was taking its toll on John. It was not merely idle gossip that he was drinking rather heavily, it was obvious to his friends who were in his presence. Since I rarely imbibed, I didn't see it myself at first.

"Over the ensuing months and years, the reports of his alcoholism became more numerous and more substantiated. He continued to have a good medical practice and no questions were ever raised about his being an excellent physician and surgeon. But his personal life became less manageable and his self-discipline eroded as if an avalanche had inundated him.

"At first I thought it was because Sally had left him, but by now I had come to realize that John's marriage to Sally had been based more on outward appearances than on true, heartfelt feelings. And in our conversations, I came to sense that what this dear friend of mine needed more than anything else was someone to truly love who would also truly love him. That's when he found Dorothy Carolyn Riggs, a young nurse at Bulloch County Hospital where they both worked. I never believed in love at first sight until I saw them together. So I wasn't surprised when they married a short time later, especially after meeting Dot and seeing how much she really loved my good friend.

"However, I began to see less of John and his new bride shortly after this, due to my increased activities at Georgia Southern College followed by three years studying for my doctorate in Chapel Hill and a year in England. It was during my work in Chapel Hill that I developed a stomach disorder and was advised to have a complete medical examination at the Duke Clinic. Tests did not indicate that there was any major difficulty, only that the tension of completing my doctorate caused some complications.

"During our year in England, I had recurring problems with my stomach and my wife insisted I have it looked into. A radiologist confirmed from a G.I. series that I had a large duodenal ulcer and three craters from former ulcers that appeared to have healed. Since we were leaving England shortly, he suggested I see a good doctor immediately upon my return to the states. So I called Dr. John the day after we got home.

"I was slightly taken aback by John's appearance when I walked into his office. He seemed to have aged more than I expected and his face was a bit ashen. While I could tell he hadn't been drinking, I sensed there was something else going on.

"But his mood was quite jovial and before long we were catching up to where we had left off almost five years earlier. What should have been a half hour check-up turned into an almost two hour gabfest. His nurse, Dallas Cason, had to come in twice to remind John that he had an office filled with impatient patients. John finally told me he would have to keep a close watch on my stomach problems and if my duodenal ulcer started hemorrhaging, it might require surgery. This necessitated my visiting his office quite frequently in the weeks and months ahead.

"It became a joke among John's office staff that when I had an appointment, they knew to extend the period of time because John and I enjoyed the visits to such an extent that our conversations were more often much longer than the medical consultation.

"Again, rumors are not very safe foundations upon which to arrive at decisions or judgments. There was now abundant talk around town of John's 'drinking too much' and appearing at social gatherings and sometimes at the hospital under the influence of alcohol. There were also stories about his wife drinking too much too often. I was aware of these remarks and observed him closely when in his office for my regular appointments. I never detected that he was under the influence of alcohol at any time.

"Having heard so often the remarks about his deteriorating physical condition, I could only be aware of any changes that I detected in his personality and mannerisms. The only thing I noticed about his physical appearance was some weight gain and at times the excessive water in and dilation of the eyes.

"It was more than a year or so later that the pains started again in my stomach and John found evidence that my ulcer was beginning to hemorrhage. He put me into the hospital for two weeks of observation, hoping to stop the hemorrhaging with medication. He always believed that surgery should be the last resort.

"While John was observing me, I was also able to observe him more closely during this period of hospitalization. When he would come by to check on me, I could not detect alcohol. Evidence pointed to the fact that he was now involved with drugs. I knew nothing about drugs. However, his pattern of behavior during the evening rounds made it evident he was taking something that had the effect of a sedative because in the morning rounds he appeared full of energy. This was not the John Mooney I had known most of my life.

"At the start of my second week of observation, John suddenly stopped making his rounds. I heard he was out of town at a medical convention and thought it strange he hadn't told me about it. At week's end, Dr. Bird Daniel came by to say the hemorrhaging had basically stopped and he was releasing me. I felt a bit better physically but rather confused about John's behavior.

"After leaving the hospital, my curiosity got the better of me so I dropped by John's office. Dallas confirmed he was out of town at a medical convention and apologized that I had not been informed. When I asked for the date he would be returning, Dallas hesitated for a moment before saying she wasn't sure. Knowing her to be a very efficient nurse, I sensed she wasn't telling me the whole truth.

"So I decided to pay a visit to John's house. I found Dot there all by herself. I could tell she had been drinking. It was a hot summer day and she said Honey and Bill Bowen had taken her three boys with them to their beach house on St. Simons Island for a few days. When I asked about John, Dot also hesitated. Then her eyes filled with tears. Perhaps because she knew John and I were very close friends or perhaps because she needed a friend herself at that moment to confide in, she suddenly broke down and told me how serious her husband's drinking and drugging had gotten.

"She said he had been going off to detox at various treatment facilities, mainly fancy resort places that cost a lot of money and did little good. She said Dallas had been covering up for him to help keep his medical practice going. I promised to keep all this to myself which made her feel more comfortable. But I left the house more confused than ever. I realized I had stepped into a world I knew absolutely nothing about. Certainly I wanted to help but I had no idea where to begin.

"I really don't believe it was my deep concern about John's welfare that caused it, but a few weeks later I awoke at home with the worst pains in my stomach I had ever experienced. I reached for the phone to call John's office and then hesitated. It was the first time in all the years we had known each other that I even had the slightest doubt about my good friend's medical abilities. Then after a moment I said to myself—if John is sober, everything will be fine. If he's not, maybe I'll have to find another doctor.

"So I called his office. He was not only sober, but I could tell he was clear-headed and clear-thinking. He told me to come right to the hospital since it sounded like my condition might require surgery.

"While dressing to leave, I noticed that my wife Addie had a very worried look on her face. It appeared to be more than just her concern about my possible surgery. She took my hand and asked if I planned to let Dr. Mooney operate on me. I knew right away why she asked. She had heard all the rumors, all the gossip. That's when I told her the same thing I had told many others in our community—that I would rather have Dr. John Mooney operate on me drunk than some other doctors operate on me sober. And as I said it, I realized that I really meant it.

"The surgery was a success and I have never had another pain in my stomach since then. But once again John wasn't around to release me from the hospital. A few days before my scheduled discharge, Dallas came by to see me. She knew about my conversation with Dot and told me in confidence that John was off on another bout with alcohol and drugs. She went on to say she had just located a special drug hospital in Lexington, Kentucky, she really believed could help him. She asked that if there were any way I could get through to him, she would be deeply grateful as would his entire family.

"A few weeks later I was due for a check-up on my surgery. I called to find that John was back at his office and would see me the following day. He looked terrible when I arrived and spoke only a few words which was most unusual. He always used his joviality to cover up his down periods.

"I wanted to ask where he had been, why he seemed to be trying to kill himself, why he couldn't simply stop his drinking and drugging. But he sensed my intentions and never gave me the chance. He simply told me the surgery came out well and that I didn't have to see him in his office for at least another six months. Then he went to check on another patient and I felt like I had been completely brushed off.

"It was more than a month later when Dallas phoned to tell me John had admitted himself into the detoxification ward at Central of Georgia Hospital in Savannah. That's when I decided to have my first real confrontation with a man I still loved and admired. I knew I could no longer just stand by and watch him die right in front of my eyes."

The Nancy Hanks was just pulling into the Atlanta train depot. Jack came out of his reverie and glanced at his watch. It wasn't quite 12:30 p.m. The train was twenty minutes early. It would give Jack more time to talk to Dr. Van Buren before seeing his friend John.

On his way to the hospital in a taxi, he began to feel a slight tinge of regret about coming to Atlanta without giving it more thought. He not only hadn't figured out yet what to say to John about his problems, but he also wasn't sure how to break some very bad news to him—news he received from Dallas just before leaving.

John's mother had been rushed to the hospital in critical condition early that same morning. The troubled physician had always been her pride and joy, and she worried about him constantly ever since her husband passed away. Before lapsing into unconsciousness at the hospital, Mrs. Sally Mooney requested that her son's picture be placed on the table next to her bed. Just how do you deliver that kind of news to a man who is already deeply troubled?

Jack tried scribbling down a few notes to pull his thoughts together, but the bumpy cab ride made it almost impossible. So the university professor who had a very deep faith simply blessed himself and left it all in the hands of his Creator.

The letter from Nurse Dallas was the pass Jack needed to be ushered without delay into Dr. Van Buren's office on the first floor of the hospital. He appeared to be a very kind and gracious man in his early seventies who reminded the professor of John's late father. But Dr. Van Buren was also a very frank man. He got right to the point.

"I can see you are the kind of person I would certainly like to have for a friend, Dr. Averitt," he said. "But I must be honest with you. I've learned that John has been addicted to alcohol and a variety of drugs for some years now. The prognosis for recovery from a combination of these substances is not positive. And there is even less hope when the addict is a physician. I think you are working with a lost man."

Once again those words—"a lost man." Hearing them from an esteemed physician gave Jack pause . . . but only for a moment. Without sounding argumentative, he told Dr. Van Buren that he recognized the truth of his statements and that he knew very little about medical science and even less about addiction.

"But I have faith that God heals," he said very softly. "And I don't believe that Dr. Mooney has to be an exception to that."

For a moment, Dr. Van Buren appeared lost for words. Then he smiled very warmly and said, "Let's go see John."

They took the elevator to the third floor and walked down a long corridor, past a busy nurses' station, to a room near the very end. Dr. Van Buren explained they were on the detoxification ward. When he opened the door and entered, Jack was almost overwhelmed by the stench of ether. At least that's what he thought it was. The doctor explained they had been giving John oral doses of something called paraldehyde to prevent him from going into delirium tremens, commonly called the DTs in the world of alcoholism. Delirium tremens is a mental disturbance characterized by confusion, disordered speech, hallucinations, and frenzied excitement caused by the prolonged use of alcoholic liquors.

Paraldehyde, which has the pungent smell of ether, is a colorless flammable liquid used to treat the DTs. Although horrible tasting, it calms the alcoholic and produces sleep for up to twelve hours with no muscle, heart, or respiratory depression. This medicine has since been replaced by safer and more effective medicines for the treatment of alcoholism and other nervous disorders.

What Jack saw lying in the bed was something he later described as "a pathetic sight." John needed a shave, was missing his dental bridge and his glasses, and looked like a bum who had been dragged in off the street. Still, when the physician saw his old friend approach, his face filled with anger and he snarled, "How can I get you off my damn back!"

Jack responded with a warm smile. "I don't break pledges. I told you in Savannah I was willing to walk the last mile with you and we still have five thousand two hundred and eighty feet to go."

John turned his face away. That's when Dr. Van Buren approached his bedside.

"I explained to Dr. Averitt the same thing I told you, John," he said, "that I think you're a lost cause. But your friend won't believe me. You should be very grateful to have someone like Dr. Averitt on your side, someone outside your family who has taken such an interest in you.

"Listen to him, John. He may not know the way, but somehow I believe he's going to find it. Listen to him, John, and follow his advice. It might be the only road you have left to travel."

Dr. Van Buren patted his patient on the arm and left. After a long moment, John turned his head back and stared up at his friend. He forced a slight smirk, trying hard not to reveal his toothless gums, and said, "Okay, Dr. Averitt. Start working your magic."

Then they both laughed. Jack reached out his hand and John

shook it. The professor said, "The first thing I'm going to do is get you all cleaned up. I'll be back here in a few minutes."

With that he left the hospital and walked to a nearby drugstore. He purchased a razor, shaving cream, a comb, and a brush. John's glasses and dental bridge would have to wait for another day. When he came back, he washed the physician's face and combed his hair. As he lathered him up and began to shave him, he could see the expression on his friend's face slowly change. It could have been the first touch of hope in a long time or possibly a momentary bit of peace and contentment. Whatever it was, it was good to see and gave Jack the courage he needed to say some things that needed to be said.

He told this once highly skilled physician how much he had admired him as a youngster for his intellectual and musical abilities, how he was his hero growing up, that everyone in Statesboro still recognized his skill as a great surgeon, and how his wife and children still loved him and prayed for his recovery.

He went on to emphasize that the John Mooney he had known for most of his life had to be restored to his proper place in society where he would once again be a contributing force in improving the quality of life for his family, his friends, and his community.

"But I think you'll agree with me, John," he concluded, "that's going to take some work. And you've become one of the most undisciplined individuals I have ever encountered. However, I believe you have the God-given ability to change all that by first finding your complete independence from alcohol and drugs. I'd like to return in a few days and discuss all that with you. I'm sure we can find some better ways for you to lick your addiction, if you don't mind my saying so."

Jack was still thinking about the drug hospital in Lexington, Kentucky, that the physician had walked out of after less than a week. However, he didn't feel like this was the right time to bring it up. So he didn't.

John simply nodded. He never said a word all the while his friend was shaving off his whiskers. Seeing the calmness that had come over him, Jack wondered whether he should break the news about his mother or wait for another time. But what if a nurse or an orderly—someone he really didn't know—found out and told him, he thought. No, it's better if he hears it from a friend.

So, after wiping the remaining shaving cream from John's face, he grabbed his friend's hand and explained as calmly as he could about his mother being taken to the hospital.

"How is she?" the physician asked very quietly as tears began to well up in his eyes.

Jack said as far as he knew, she was in very good care. He promised to find out more upon his return home and call him right away. He also promised to contact John's ophthalmologist and get him a new pair of glasses. As they shook hands very warmly, Jack could see the gratitude on his friend's more pleasant-looking countenance.

Before leaving the hospital, the professor gave the head nurse his phone number and asked her to call if any problems arose. Then he just managed to catch the 6 p.m. train back to Statesboro.

Dr. Averitt kept a very busy schedule over the next several days. He called John in Atlanta each morning to tell him his mother was resting comfortably. Then he would head off to Georgia Southern College to teach class until 4:30 p.m. On his way home, he would stop by Lee Street to fill Dot in on her husband's progress and try to buoy her spirits.

"Each time I paid her a visit," the professor later wrote in his journal, "she would tell me how she was willing to do anything to help her husband. The problem was, I began to sense she might need as much help as John.

"There was always the smell of beer throughout the house, her eyes were usually glassy and her speech generally a bit slurred. However, I knew that anything I said would not be well received. So I said nothing. All it did was cause more confusion in my life."

It was about 11 a.m. on Friday, July 3, when the professor dropped by John's office to get more information from Dallas about the

Lexington drug facility. He planned to discuss with his friend that weekend in Atlanta the possibility of his returning there for the full treatment program. Before leaving, Jack called the hospital to let the still-recovering physician know when he would be arriving. He was shocked when the head nurse told him that "Dr. Mooney disappeared from the hospital about an hour ago and we don't know where he went."

Jack demanded to know how such a thing could have happened and why he was not informed. The nurse apologized, explaining she and her staff were very busy at the time treating some newly arrived patients. She said she learned that Dr. Mooney had called George Muse's Clothing Store in Atlanta and they brought him a suit, shoes, socks, a shirt and tie, and a Panama straw hat. Then he called a cab and left before anyone could stop him.

"I was so exasperated by it all," Dr. Averitt later wrote, "that I was almost inclined to just let it go, to stop trying to play God. But then I saw the despairing look on the face of Dallas Cason. She had gone to such great lengths to help save this man and I hadn't yet gone the full mile that I had promised him."

So the professor reached for the Atlanta telephone directory on the nearby bookshelf and began checking the yellow pages to find a private detective agency.

John Mooney well remembered his thinking that day, and he often shared it with friends later in his life.

"My intentions were to go back to Statesboro to see my mother," he explained. "But I didn't have much money left after paying for all those new clothes. And as I walked through the streets of the city, I began to get very nervous and confused, almost panicking at times. I thought I might have enough for a train ticket, but then I would also need something to calm my nerves. I had to make a choice."

The physician wound up checking into the Henry Grady Hotel in Atlanta, only two steps removed from a flophouse. He had purchased three quarts of bourbon whiskey, which he carried in a brown paper bag. That's where Dr. John Mooney Jr. went on his last bender—and it was a dilly.

"I got insanely drunk," he recalled, "gulping down big water glasses filled with straight bourbon. I would pass out, come to, drink some more, and pass out again. It was almost like I wanted to drink myself to death.

"Then, sometime around two o'clock on the morning of July 4, 1959, two men came bursting into my room. They wore dark suits with gray hats. Somehow I knew it was the law, probably because they didn't take off their hats. They told me that Sheriff Howell from Statesboro sent them to arrest me. I knew my goose was finally cooked.

"Still, I asked them if I could take another drink before they took me away and they agreed. So I poured myself a really big glassful and downed it. Then I looked at the level of the booze in the bottle and marked it on the label with my fingernail. I always did this because I never want somebody else drinking from my bottle when I wasn't there. I planned on coming back and finishing it myself. That's how insanely drunk I was at the time."

What John didn't know at that point was that his good friend, Jack Averitt, had set in motion a series of events that were to eventually save his life.

Jack had hired a private detective in Atlanta named Colonel Alston. He and his partner tracked the physician to the Henry Grady Hotel by that evening, but could do nothing since they didn't have a warrant to take him into custody. They simply sat outside the hotel in their car to make sure he didn't leave.

Meanwhile, the dedicated professor went to see Dot to bring her up to date and to ask her advice. John's two sisters happened to be there. They had just come from Bulloch County Hospital and were talking about the seriousness of their mother's illness. When Jack explained their brother's plight and asked if they had any thoughts about what to do, the older sister, Mary Lind, insisted that "we just forget that John Mooney ever lived."

Dot began to cry and the younger sister, Sarah, got very angry. After a moment, Dot took Jack's hand and pleaded with him to do whatever he felt was in her husband's best interest. She trusted him implicitly. Sarah said the same thing. Mary Lind said nothing else.

The professor hurried home and called John's attorney, George Johnston. He suggested they file a lunacy warrant in order to take the physician into custody and bring him back to the Bulloch County Jail. At that point, they might possibly be able to talk him into some further treatment. But they would need a judge to sign the warrant.

Once again Dr. Jack Averitt's reputation and respect in the community greased the wheels of justice. He phoned his friend Probate Court Judge Robert Mikell and explained the situation; the lunacy warrant was drawn up and signed before midnight. Sheriff Howell then sent a copy of it by Western Union to the Atlanta Police Department. At 2 a.m., two Atlanta detectives showed up at the Henry Grady and John Mooney was soon on his way back to Statesboro—in handcuffs.

While he knew his addiction now had complete control over his life, the physician seemed oblivious to the other problems piling up on him. Federal narcotics agents had been in his office the day before, attempting to trace prescriptions he had written for drugs using false names or the names of patients who never received them. Dallas had told Dr. Averitt, but they decided to keep it from John until other matters were settled.

Jack had heard from George Johnston that it was only a matter of time before the Feds had enough evidence to bring felony drug charges against the impaired physician, so they had to work fast if they were to help him escape that fate.

It was feared that John might relapse into the DTs again if he were locked up in the Bulloch County Jail. So instead, he was taken to the security ward at St. Joseph's Hospital in Savannah and once again administered oral doses of paraldehyde.

Two days later, on Tuesday morning, July 7, Mrs. Sally Mooney passed away. Her son, who still had not seen her during her critical period at the hospital, was filled with remorse. He went into a deep depression and the hospital staff was ordered to keep a close watch on him. He kept insisting that he be allowed to attend his mother's funeral.

The tending physician at St. Joseph's gave his okay provided someone stayed close to the depressed surgeon at all times. Since the lunacy warrant was still in effect, John was accompanied to the funeral home and later to the cemetery by a deputy sheriff. This embarrassed him no end. Even though he was filled with guilt and knew deep inside that all this was his own fault, he once again turned his anger on Jack Averitt for filing the lunacy warrant. The fact that this man was still walking that mile beside him seemed to make no difference. It's important to note that the disease of alcoholism and drug abuse fosters character defects and shortcomings that cause addicts to blame others for their problems rather than blame themselves regardless of the situation.

In addition to the deep remorse John felt over his mother's death, he could hardly bear the pain of seeing Dot at the funeral, especially knowing the fear she must have felt about the unstable future before them—not knowing how or when or whether there would be peace and harmony in their home and in their lives. So they said little except that they loved each other and hoped somehow God wouldn't let them down. Despite all that had happened and all that was to happen, the one thing that John and Dot had never lost was their faith in God.

Dr. Jack Averitt was convinced by now that nothing but the harshest treatment for his addiction problems would bring his friend to his senses. And he still believed, as did Dallas Cason, the best such treatment could be found in Lexington, Kentucky—not just at the hospital he walked away from, but at the prison itself. And if there was something that could be worked out before the hammer of the federal narcotics agents came down on John, it might prove to be the best solution all the way around.

George Johnston agreed. So did Sheriff Howell and another friend of Dr. Averitt's, the local district attorney. Together they met with Superior Court Judge J. L. Renfroe in his chambers at 11 a.m. on July 10. They explained the problem in every detail, describing Dr. John Mooney's warts as well as his assets, his abilities as well as his addictions, his major contributions together with his drawbacks. They also mentioned that federal narcotics agents were close on his trail. They concluded by asking Judge Renfroe, a kindly man in his late sixties, to "sentence" the impaired physician to the United States Narcotics Prison in Lexington so that he could be treated for his addictions and hopefully return to society the man he once was—a major contributive citizen of Statesboro.

Although the judge knew all about John's problems from his many discussions over the years with his friends and colleagues in town, he was very reluctant at first to take such drastic action. However, once he heard about the government's narcotics agents looking to hang this hometown doctor, Judge Renfroe began to soften his opposition to the request before him. Also, he had been at Mrs. Mooney's funeral since she and her husband were among his close circle of friends. And he once admired their son, whom he knew to be an excellent doctor and a credit to his community before his malady set in. So, in the end, he agreed with Dr. Averitt and the others that this was a man worth saving.

For the process to go forward, however, someone would have to bring drug felony charges against John and someone would have to give testimony as to those charges so that he could be legitimately sentenced to the drug prison. Sheriff Howell agreed to bring the charges, and Jack reluctantly agreed to testify since no one else would.

Dot was at her husband's bedside in St. Joseph's security ward the next morning when Jack and the others explained to the now totally beaten physician the deal that had been worked out with Judge Renfroe. Every bone in John's body wanted to object. The crazy man living in his brain kept telling him he could do it on his own—that going to prison was way over the top. But then his heart told him there was no other way out. It was time to pay the piper. He looked around at these men who he knew were on his side and told them he was willing to do whatever they thought best.

Jack Averitt remembered seeing the tears rolling down Dot's face. She was holding tight to both of her husband's hands as if unwilling to let go. That's when the professor nudged the sheriff, John's attorney, and the district attorney. They all left the room to let the couple digest everything that just happened. Dot later shared with friends what went through her mind that morning.

"I kept thinking how we did almost everything together. We walked together. We laughed together. We played with our boys together. We cried together. We stayed in bed together. And we drank and took drugs together. We had a marriage of trying to be together whenever we could.

"That can be good, but it can also be bad. And when it came to the alcohol and drugs, it was bad. Very bad. I thought for a moment that because we did so much together, maybe we should go to prison together. I said that to John, that I would be willing to go wherever he went. He kissed me and hugged me and then laughed, saying who would take care of the boys. So I promised him I would do my best and be there for him when he came home."

The next morning, a very confused and nervous physician stood before Judge J. L. Renfroe to hear his fate:

"Dr. John Mooney, you have been convicted of a drug felony and I hereby sentence you to two years in the Georgia State Prison in Reidsville. However, I do not think you are a criminal. I believe you are a very sick man. And I am convinced by your record that you need treatment for your addictions. Therefore, I am going to probate that sentence provided you enter the United

States Narcotics Prison and Hospital in Lexington, Kentucky and stay there until the day you are pronounced cured and officially released."

While Judge Renfroe was speaking, so was the crazy man still in John's head. He wouldn't let up. He kept telling the physician he should hate this judge who claims to be his friend. How can he be when he's just committed such a grave injustice. The crazy man in his brain was always so convincing that John usually did his bidding—like tell this judge off. Tell him he doesn't know what he's talking about. Some years later the physician shared with friends what he actually said to the judge after he imposed the sentence.

"Your Honor," he remarked, "I appreciate what you are trying to do. I believe you want to do what you think is best for me. But I've never stepped foot in your courtroom before this. I feel I deserve a break. I want to tell you as truthfully as I can that I have learned my lesson. I've been through some terrible experiences in the last few weeks.

"I know what I was doing was wrong. So I'm going to get into a program somewhere and get somebody to help me with this drinking and drugging because I'm not going to do it anymore. And I'd like to stay out here and prove to you that I don't have to go to either place. I've gone as far as I could go and still survived. Now I'm ready to do something about it."

At that point, Judge Renfroe's face turned a bit red. He glared down at the physician and replied rather sternly.

"John, there may be something wrong with your ears. I don't think you heard me. You're either going to Reidsville or you're going to Lexington. Which is it?"

After a moment, John also turned a little red-faced, blushing with shame. He replied rather humbly, "I'll take Lexington, Your Honor."

Before leaving the courtroom in the hands of a deputy sheriff,

John approached Jack Averitt. He wanted to apologize for the lack of appreciation he showed at times for his deep friendship, for not understanding the need for the lunacy warrant, for getting so angry with him the day of his mother's funeral, and, most important, for saving his life. Jack could never forget that brief conversation and later noted in his journal some of the words his good friend said to him:

"I can't tell you how much I regret letting my mother down. She had always insisted that I have the best of everything, especially when it came to academic training. At a time when perhaps I could have helped her the most, while she lay sick in the hospital, I wasn't there for her. I will have to live with that for the rest of my life."

On Monday, July 13, Dr. John Mooney Jr. went back to Lexington, Kentucky, only this time it wasn't to the hospital. It was to the prison. And he didn't drive there in his 1956 white Ford Thunderbird with its red convertible top. He flew there with a deputy sheriff, who accompanied him right up to the front gate of the ominous federal correctional facility. Before departing, the physician remembered the deputy saying to him quite bluntly, "Judge Renfroe said to tell you that if you don't cooperate with the authorities here and you try to leave this place, I'll be back at this gate to pick you up and take you directly to the state prison in Reidsville, where you'll do hard time for the next two years."

John turned and stared up at the high walls. That's when the realization finally struck that he would be here for as long as it would take him to get well.

CHAPTER ELEVEN

More Will Be Revealed

ALTHOUGH MENTALLY AND PHYSICALLY EXHAUSTED, JOHN Mooney got very little sleep his first night in prison. The strange and eerie sounds coming from the cell block, along with the unending voices in his head, kept him tossing and turning on his hard, thin mattress until the first signs of daylight began to creep into his small cubicle.

His first thought as he pushed himself erect was, "If this is bad, I can't imagine what it must be like in Reidsville."

His next thought was, "I hope Dot and the boys will be all right without me." Then he smirked at himself, saying aloud, "Sure, she's going to miss a lousy husband and they're going to miss a lousy father."

John didn't realize it at first, but this was another sign of the self-honesty that was finally beginning to emerge inside him, the kind of rigorous honesty he had tried to avoid most of his life by taking another drink or another drug. But now he was clean and sober, or at least at the very beginning of recovery, and he was slowly realizing that this kind of self-honesty would be essential to any long-lasting solution.

He looked down at the number stamped across the front of his gray prison uniform. "Dr. 58520" was coming to understand that no alcoholic or drug addict can be helped unless he first admits to his innermost self what he is. As a physician, John was used to diagnosing the ills of others. But addicts must diagnose themselves. For the disease of alcoholism or drug addiction only really exists when the addict sees it and admits it to himself.

"If someone had asked me just a few weeks before I entered prison if I had any real trouble in my life," he once admitted, "I would have said no, I don't have any major problems. I'm just sick, and if I don't stop doing what I'm doing, I could wind up in some serious trouble.

"It wasn't until the felony drug conviction that I started to realize I had some real problems in my life, and had had them for some time. The truth is, I had already been obtaining illegal drugs and using them by the carloads long before this all came down. I was already in deep trouble without being honest enough to admit it, especially to myself.

"The only important thing for me at the time was not getting found out. Don't let anybody know about it and everything will be okay. When you have the kind of ego and pride I have, someone has to use a sledgehammer to make you face the truth about yourself. Being sentenced to the narcotics prison was my sledgehammer."

He stood up and stretched, then walked slowly to the barred window of his cell. It was already dark when he was incarcerated the night before, so there was little he could see outside. Now as he glanced through the window, he noticed the green pastures just beyond the prison wall and a herd of Angus cattle grazing contentedly in the early morning sunlight. He snickered at himself once again as he thought, "Look at all those so-called dumb animals gamboling free in that meadow out there. And look at me, a so-called smart doctor with all my medical degrees, locked up in here with no freedom at all. Now that's something to really think about."

A shrill whistle broke into his thoughts. Then his cell door suddenly rolled open as a loud voice shouted, "Step out for a countdown."

Two uniformed guards paraded down the gangway past his cell without saying a word. After a moment, there was another whistle. All the prisoners turned and headed off toward a nearby stairwell. John simply followed them, assuming it was time for breakfast.

As he entered the prison dining hall, John started to realize there was something different this time about being back in Lexington. He had no panicky feelings in his gut. And the people seemed to have changed. They appeared to be friendlier. Some greeted him and patted him on the back. Even the big, black-bearded guy that he had a run-in with over the saltshaker came up to him and said, "John, glad to see you back."

Some years later, the physician told a group of friends that he had suddenly become aware that he was finally facing reality and was beginning to accept it. For some strange reason, he was even comfortable with it. Those fellows he once called "bums" and was afraid of the first time around now seemed more like him than the elite circle of acquaintances he had back in Statesboro.

"I had no idea how far down the road I had traveled with my addiction until I confronted it there in the narcotics prison," he said. "I was one of them and they were one of me. Like practically everyone there, I hadn't just hit the bottom—I kicked the bottom out and kept on going down.

"It was like that old story of the three umpires who were arguing one day about balls and strikes. The first one said, 'I call them like I see them.' The next one said, 'I call them like they are.' The last one said, 'They ain't nothing until I call them.'

"I finally saw my real problem and called it what it was—total powerlessness over any and all kinds of drugs."

As John was finishing his breakfast, a guard wearing sergeant's stripes approached to inform him he had a nine o'clock meeting scheduled with the prison psychiatric board. So he left his cup of lukewarm coffee and followed the sergeant to the office of Dr. Daniel C. Beittel, a psychologist in his late forties who proceeded to give him a Rorschach test.

More popularly known as the inkblot test, it was created by Swiss psychologist Hermann Rorschach in 1921 to examine a person's personality characteristics and emotional functioning. A psychologist records the subject's perceptions of inkblots and analyzes them using psychological interpretation.

The test has been employed to detect underlying thought disorder, especially in patients who are reluctant to describe their thinking processes openly. The Rorschach test is the second most widely used test by members of the Society of Personality Assessment and is requested by more than 80 percent of clinical psychiatrists.

"I've had so many Rorschach tests," John recalled, "I can almost take them without looking at the inkblots. Dr. Beittel also told me he had stacks of my medical records from all the treatment facilities I had gone to over the years and said he would be comparing his findings with those in the various reports. I forgot I had signed a waiver to allow them to see all these reports, most of which I had never seen myself."

John then spent another hour or so answering questions from a panel of three other doctors, all of whom seemed quite friendly and supportive. One in particular, Doctor James D. Hawthorne, expressed a rather deep interest in the case of "58520," and said he would like to spend some time talking with him at a later date.

While the Statesboro surgeon thought the meeting went well, he would have been very disappointed and possibly a bit angry had he read the initial report Dr. Beittel prepared for the board. More than a year later, John saw what the psychologist had written about him:

The patient is a 49-year-old white, married, male physician who has been placed under the care of Dr. Hawthorne. My initial findings are in essential agreement with Dr.

Hawthorne, with the possible exception that I see this patient as a severe character disorder with very little anxiety and relatively un-amenable to therapy at the present time, despite his high intelligence and physician status.

He is essentially here to beat a Federal rap which was dropped on the circumstances that he be sent here to complete a Hospital Treatment Program, and he is very interested in getting out of here in the minimum amount of time with very little involvement. He has had previous psychiatric contacts, including admissions to Silver Hill and elsewhere and these have all eventually resulted in relapse to narcotics addiction. The patient does not seem in any danger to himself and it is anticipated he will relapse to the use of narcotics after his discharge.

I would suggest minimum criteria for this patient and would expect him to make a conforming sort of hospital adjustment.

The "minimum criteria" meant John was to be transferred from his prison cell to a dormitory at the hospital, where he could mingle with other alcoholics and drug addicts and attend more therapy sessions without having to be in the company of a prison guard.

Meanwhile on the home front, things weren't going all that well, even though family, friends, and neighbors did what they could to help. As the days, weeks, and months passed, many in Statesboro wondered when Dr. Mooney would be getting out of prison, whether he would be a changed man after his time away, and how his family was faring during these stressful times.

"I had never been lonelier in my whole life with John being away in prison," Dot remembered when she thought about those days. "Even though I had my boys around me, I always had this fear and dread inside, not knowing how we would get by and what it would be like once John came home. I was so dependent on him. Still, I tried my best to carry on like we were a normal family."

In sharing her experiences during that dark period in her life, Dot once jokingly said there was only one thing that made her life a bit easier with her husband being away. She didn't have to worry about him burning down the house.

"John was a very heavy smoker and even more so when he drank," she explained. "I was always afraid that when he drank too much, his lit cigarette might somehow set the place on fire. So I would sit up until late at night to keep an eye on him.

"One night he was drinking and smoking in the parlor. I was so tired I had to go to bed. That's when his cigarette fell on my favorite carpet and set it on fire. He started stumbling around to put it out and woke me up. Smoke from the burning carpet filled the whole downstairs of the house. After the fire was out, we had a furious argument. I was especially mad because he knew how much I loved that carpet.

"So the next day he comes home with a brand new fire-resistant carpet. He says I could stop worrying because the new carpet can't catch fire. But I still tried to stay awake when he smoked and drank so he wouldn't set the bed on fire. Once he went off to prison I could finally get some sleep."

But with her husband gone, Dot had to make some serious decisions about her own actions and her own addictions. As she once shared, "Demerol and alcohol used to calm my fears, but I decided with my husband not home, I shouldn't drink liquor if I was to be a good mother for my children. So I just drank beer. I always heard that you couldn't be a real alcoholic if you only drank beer. That's crazy thinking, but then . . . I guess I became as crazy as my husband and wouldn't admit it to myself or anybody else."

Dot was now visiting her mother more frequently, and Myrtis and Dot's brother, Arthur James, always made sure she went home with plenty of food. Some old friends from church would also drop by on occasion to leave some fresh fruits and vegetables and goodies for the boys, saying they were only doing what Dot and John would do for someone else.

Even most of John's old friends still stuck by him during this uncertain period in his life. Ike Minkovitz, for example, the Jewish businessman, signed a few more notes at the bank to keep the mortgage payments on the Lee Street house current. Attorney George Johnston continued to fend off the IRS, and Dr. Jack Averitt kept in touch with his friend through frequent correspondence.

Still, while John was in the process of getting well, Dot—despite her feeble attempts to control her addiction to alcohol and drugs—was getting sicker.

"I was always going to quit tomorrow," she would often tell close friends. "But then I'd get very nervous and feel a spell coming on, so I would have a few beers. And it was never a few beers.

"One Sunday morning I got up to take my children to Sunday school and I found myself literally shaking so much I couldn't get dressed. I went into the kitchen, opened the refrigerator, and drank three bottles of beer right in a row. As I opened the fourth, I started to cry. Drinking all this beer was not what I wanted to do. I sat down and began to sob. I knew I was out of control, but I couldn't stop.

"My children came into the kitchen to see if I was ready for church and they saw me crying. Instead of responding with love and understanding, I got angry and yelled at them to get out of the kitchen. I understood why I was so angry. I hated myself and was embarrassed that my sons saw their mother in such a state."

Dot took her children to Sunday school that morning in her bathrobe. She dropped them off and went back home to have another beer. She didn't remember going back to pick them up or how she took care of them the rest of that day.

"I was so upset with myself that I needed someone to talk to, someone close. So the following afternoon I asked my dear friend, Honey Bowen, to watch my boys so I could ride over to Jimps and speak with my brother, Arthur James, whom I loved and respected so much.

"I poured my heart out to him about the loneliness, the hurt, the heartache, the fear, and all those terrible feelings going on inside me. I knew my brother loved me too, so what I expected from him was some comfort and understanding. What I got instead was disappointing and hurtful and it made me a little angry. Of course, I know now what I got was the unvarnished truth."

Her soft-spoken, rugged-looking older brother, who also was a war hero, handed his sister his handkerchief to wipe the tears from her eyes and to blow her running nose. Then he said, trying not to sound too judgmental, "Dot, you're an alcoholic. You don't have any business drinking, especially with John away and you having to take care of those boys of yours. You have to stop. You already have a lot of trouble in your life. You don't need any more."

The distraught mother drove home that night and sat in her car for almost an hour before going into the house. She knew her sons were already asleep at Honey's, so she decided not to disturb them. She just couldn't get her brother's words out of her mind.

Dot went into the kitchen, opened the refrigerator, and stared at the shelf filled with bottles of cold beer. Then she closed the door, got some writing paper and a pen from a cabinet drawer, and sat down at the kitchen table. She wrote John another letter that night, only this time for some reason she decided to be as honest as she could be about her circumstances without trying to worry her husband too much.

She admitted to him that she was still drinking—but only beer—and really and truly wanted to stop. She told him what her brother had said and how it affected her. Attempting to hold the pen steady, Dot asked John if the treatment program in Lexington was showing him any way to break his addiction, and if so, to please write and let her know. This country girl, filled with so much apprehension, was being as truthful as her heart would let her to this man she still loved so deeply and needed so desperately in her life.

In writing that letter, Dot Mooney had no idea she was starting to find what her husband was finding in prison—that touch of self-honesty addicts need to emerge from the morass holding them hostage. However, when Dot finished the letter, she needed another bottle of beer to help her sleep. She took two more into her bedroom with her.

While this confused and lonely mother was trying to be honest with herself and with her husband, she was not being honest with her children. She never told them that their father was in prison, nor did anyone else in the family or among their friends. Dot told them the usual story of their dad going off to some medical conference to learn more about being a better doctor. But as the weeks and months passed, her sons began to suspect there was something she wasn't telling them, especially her oldest son.

Al Mooney was now ten years old, and as the weeks passed by, he became convinced his father was not at some drawn-out medical meeting because he had never been away this long before. It just didn't make any sense to him.

"So his going off to some doctor's conference began to fall apart for me," Al explained. "I don't know whether people were just ashamed to tell me he was in prison, or what was going on. But I guess it's something people commonly do. They don't want the kids to know everything, especially if they think it will upset them, so they just don't tell them the truth. And the truth is usually a lot less painful than all the stories a child makes up in his mind because he doesn't know the truth.

"I don't know whether my mother didn't want to tell me the truth or she just didn't know how. So you have to make up a story for yourself, and you have to make up one that can cover all the bases. Mine was that my father was dead and nobody had the guts to tell me. And I consciously remember that to this very day.

I went from being very confused to being very sure that my father was dead, but I still couldn't figure out how I was going to get the real answer.

"So even though I was sure, I kind of waited for proof one way or the other. I simply said to myself that if he were dead, I'd never see him again. But if he was alive, I'd see him someday."

Jimmy Mooney, who was nine at the time, only remembers his mother telling him, "Daddy's off at some medical thing and will be gone for a while." Since he was used to his father being away for weeks at a time, he just accepted her story.

"I honestly don't believe I even knew that he went to prison until maybe just before he came home," Jimmy said. "But I knew there was something different going on by the way my mother acted. She seemed more nervous and short-tempered at times than when my father was around.

"But still, it wasn't unusual to me that my father was away again. I only knew that when he finally did come home, he would be bringing us a whole lot of gifts because that's the way he tried to show his love for us."

On the other hand, Bobby, who was only six years old when his father was incarcerated, remembers little about him being gone, but more about his mother's trials and tribulations.

"I do recall my mother seeming to pay more attention to me than usual," Bobby explained. "I mean, I always felt close to her and knew that she loved me, but now it felt extra special.

"Also I seem to remember going a lot to Savannah with her and my brothers where I later found out she was getting electric shock treatments. She sometimes wouldn't remember how to get home and my brothers Al and Jimmy had to tell her. That's the only time I think I wondered why my daddy wasn't around to help us."

One person who *was* always around was Dallas Cason. While her boss was doing his time at the Lexington narcotics facility, Dallas remained as loyal to him and his family as she had always been.

There was no problem keeping the medical office on Siebald Street open because the Mooney estate owned the building. But because of the warning she had received from the State of Georgia Registration Board, the nurse had to be very careful about treating any patients who came by.

"But I did manage to continue collecting some old patient bills," she said, "which helped Dot meet some of her own expenses. And my good friend Jack Averitt would frequently drop by to keep me abreast of Dr. Mooney's welfare and progress with his addiction. They were writing to each other regularly."

Then something happened that rather surprised the dedicated nurse and made her think seriously about her present circumstances.

"Dr. Daniel came by the office one day," Dallas explained, "and asked if I would like to go to work for him. He said no one knew how long Dr. Mooney would be gone and that he could use someone with my skills in his practice.

"I thought at first that perhaps I should talk with my husband about it or even Dot who, even though she was Dr. Mooney's wife, I considered a very close friend. Then I realized I didn't have to do either. I just told Dr. Daniel no, that Dr. Mooney was not only my boss but also my friend, and that if there ever was a time when he needed me, it was now. So I didn't go to work for him."

Dr. Averitt wrote John periodically as well as visited Dot on a weekly basis. He would check on whatever information she had received from or about her husband, and he would share what John wrote to him.

"She seemed pleased with John's attitude and his response to treatment," the professor wrote in his journal. "We all knew that John's most difficult problem was to subordinate himself to another's leadership and become subservient to the policies that were established for him. This was in direct conflict with his usual method of action."

One particular letter Jack received from his friend pleased him immensely. It helped to convince him that John was finally on the right path. The letter read in part:

"Just like all institutions, including hospitals, colleges and military installations, everybody here castigates the food and all the restrictions as well as the people who are responsible for it. Even though griping is part of the reality of life, especially in a place like this, I've decided not to engage in it and just accept things as they are. It's better for what little sanity I have left.

"The patients in this institution seem to represent every trade, profession, social level and category of American life. I've discovered that many doctors come here but most are quickly horrified by the prospect of spending a prolonged period of time in such a place, just as I once did. So, even when faced with state and Federal court action, they leave before the doctors dismiss them, despite knowing that is worse in the eyes of most courts than not coming at all. I've heard that some of them are met at the prison gate by the FBI or Federal narcotics agents the very day they leave here.

"Frankly, I believe there is enough pressure on me from the State of Georgia to make me stay even if I wanted to or could leave. Certainly I want out of this whole mess as soon as possible, but I've discovered that the way patients here adapt themselves to procedures seems to be a major fact in their prognosis. I've learned that from the majority of patients. I've also been told by the psychiatrists here that about 80 to 85 percent of the patients have no desire to be helped at all or seriously consider a life without drugs. I don't want to be included in that percentage.

"As far as I'm concerned, I don't think I could be in a better place right now. You are on your own and get what you ask for, including medical treatments. The psychological staff cannot possibly treat everybody, so they see only those who request it. If you want, you can get complete analysis which takes several years. Some patients take it for some time and then continue as an outpatient once they're released. I believe there are other options as well which I'm looking into.

"You know that after going through all this, Jack, I really want to get well. So I must decide what option would be best for me. I will certainly let you know what I decide."

Shortly after this, Jack and his wife, Addie, left on a planned seven-week tour of Europe.

"I wasn't unable to keep in touch with John on a regular basis during this time, although I did drop him a line from each of our stops," he recorded in his journal. "However, the indication of his adjustment to the treatment and discipline seemed to be so positive that I tried not to worry about not hearing from him."

When Jack and his wife finally arrived back in Statesboro, there was a letter from John waiting for the professor. It was quite upbeat and read in part:

"Your letters from Europe were most informative. I was able to live again many of the scenes and situations which I encountered during the abnormal times when I was there. I don't believe that even war can temper the beauty of Vesuvius or Capri. Many of the places in Northern Italy I could not visit until 1943 . . . not because of the Italians. They were willing enough. But the Germans took a rather dim view of touring Americans at that time.

"Some day in the future, I hope Dot and I can tour the Continent. We will probably need to do it soon, too, as according to historical schedule, it is about due to be shot up again."

John had begun attending scheduled group therapy sessions with other drug-addicted patients and prisoners, cautiously sharing his experience about how his drug use started during the war, how it came to affect his family, his medical practice, and his entire life, and how it eventually led him to Lexington. He was also starting to meet every week or so with Dr. James Hawthorne, who had taken a particular interest in his case.

In fact, Dr. Hawthorne did a rather thorough psychiatric work-up on the incarcerated physician, using Dr. Beitell's Rorschach test results, the reports from other hospitals, and his own consultations with John. After finishing his workup, he gave his patient a copy to review and offer any comments he would like to make.

The report helped John see himself as he was and as others saw him. It also opened him up to even greater self-honesty. He kept Dr. Hawthorne's psychiatric report among his private papers until the day he passed away. Here is what it said:

"The patient is a 49-year-old white, male physician who came to this hospital for a second admission. He is married and of the Protestant faith.

"The patient admits that he has always had a tendency to excesses. He recalls that when he was in college, he suffered from a sinus condition which necessitated repeated drainage. He would look forward to his visits with the physician because the cocaine used as a topical anesthetic gave him a very pleasant sensation. He further recalls that he tended to consume alcohol in excess while in college, although not to the degree of interfering with his studies.

"During his years of medical training, he recalls that he tended to use a lot of cocaine for relief of the usual manifestations of an upper respiratory infection.

"Addiction did not become a problem until he joined the armed forces and saw considerable action in World War II. Returning home was a very trying period for the patient, as he was soon involved in a divorce from his first wife on the grounds of infidelity. They had been married for a period of 10 years. Also during this period, the patient states his father died from carcinoma of the lung, and following his father's death, his mother seemed to lose interest in living.

"He began to drink more heavily during this time and to use whatever drugs were in his medical bag. He used codeine, Pantapon and Demerol, orally and intra-muscularly, but he says he has never used a narcotic agent intravenously.

"He has been treated for varying periods up to three months in a number of private sanitaria and hospitals and has had short periods of therapy from a number of psychiatrists. He desisted from the use of all alcohol and drugs for almost one year following a course of treatment in a private sanitarium. He began using narcotics again when he sustained a fracture to one of his fingers.

"The patient is here because Georgia State authorities arrested him on a felony drug charge and basically gave him a suspended sentence provided he come here for 'the cure.' The Federal charge has been dropped and he understands that the state charge will be stricken from the records following his discharge from this hospital.

"The patient is a neat, pleasant-appearing, alert, animated, middle-aged individual. He is comfortable in the interview process and gives information freely without undue probing. Psychomotor activity is somewhat increased, but is felt to be appropriate, and there are no tics or tremors. His memory is adequate for past and recent events, and affect appears appropriate for ideation expressed.

"The patient gives the impression that much of his psychomotor activity, gestures, etc. and much of his pleasantness and friendliness are forced at the conscious level. He has feelings of inferiority which he has made a conscious effort to overcome through competition and participation in various activities.

"Intelligence is estimated as well above average. Accuracy of judgment and reasoning ability also are well above average.

"There is no evidence of phobias, serious compulsions or psychotic thought. One doubts that the patient's insight is very deep despite the fact that he speaks of feelings of inferiority, overcompensation, tendency toward excesses, etc. It is felt that his insight concerning his addiction is nil.

"The test responses on the patient's Rorschach were consistent with an hypothesis of deep conflicting need systems as follows:

"One, he is gravely anxious that he is inadequate not only as a man and as a father, but also that he is sick in some unknown or actually phobic way;

"Two, he is fearful of libidinal pressures;

"Three, he is fearful of the paradoxical boredom and lack of fulfillment of his deep succorant needs in his heavy routine of work;

"Four, he is a very intelligent person who finds himself at odds with many requirements as an important person in his community;

"Five, he probably cannot face the external super-ego in the form of older women whom he sees as 'sour' and prim.

"In summary, the Rorschach reveals that this complex person is caught in numerous pressures, driven by his high intelligence to seek fulfillment, aware at some level of his moral and ethical confusion of loyalty, needing assurance in many ways and unconsciously resenting many of the demands made upon him. His struggles sometimes made him feel worse than being lonely. They often make him feel completely alone.

"The patient is the product of an intact home. The family was of the upper social strata and there were no financial problems. The atmosphere was permissive, protected and indulgent. However, one gets the feeling that family relationships were cool. The patient was hampered in his social development due to over-protection on a physical basis. This led to feelings of inferiority which the patient has been able to handle admirably by conscious effort and self discipline.

"He has been able to establish and maintain a good surgical practice, entered actively into community, religious and medical organizations and has at times been a better than average leader. This seems to indicate a superior intelligence and a great ego. It would appear that his major downfall has been the abuse of drugs.

"There were no children born into his first marriage despite the fact that children were wanted and no physical defect could be determined. He re-married shortly after separating from his first wife. He has been able to make a good adjustment with his second wife and now has three sons.

"Sexual development appears to be 'normal.' The only sexual

problem he has ever had is that of premature ejaculation which he attributes to mild phimosis and the use of drugs. The patient has limited insight into his problems, but his superior intellect and ego strengths have allowed him to function efficiently. He has tried psychotherapy in the past and does not feel that it has helped.

"It is felt that any proposal of long-range therapy should be delayed until the patient is better motivated. He has already made a good vocational and institutional adjustment, but may push for an early discharge. His prognosis regarding his addiction must remain guarded."

Since Dr. Hawthorne saw a strong pattern of alcohol abuse in his patient's history, he strongly suggested that he start attending some meetings of AA, which was known in the prison at that time as "Addicts Anonymous." But alcoholics also attended these meetings, which were brought into the hospital several times a week by an outside group of Alcoholics Anonymous. John had heard of Alcoholics Anonymous at some of the other facilities he frequented. He had often been urged to join. But the surgeon's awareness of his addiction was limited to his dependence on narcotics, and he denied he was an alcoholic. Dr. Hawthorne's recommendation would prove instrumental in changing his patient's life, however.

The Fellowship of Alcoholics Anonymous was started in May 1935 by two desperate drunks seeking some way to stay sober. Their lives were in shambles from their addiction to booze. One was Bill Wilson, a bankrupt Wall Street investor who was in Akron, Ohio, at the time, wrapping up another failed business deal. Ready to drink again, he met through a series of fortuitous circumstances an alcoholic doctor named Robert Smith whose medical practice was in ruins.

Together, by sharing their painful drinking experiences, they found they could help each other stay sober. They came to describe the Twelve-Step recovery program they created—and which now comprises more than two million recovered alcoholics around the world—as follows:

> Alcoholics Anonymous is a fellowship of men and women who share their experience, strength and hope with each other that they may solve their common problem and help others to recover from alcoholism. The only requirement for membership is a desire to stop drinking. There are no dues or fees for AA membership. We are self-supporting through our own contributions. AA is not allied with any sect, denomination, politics, organization or institution; does not engage in any controversy; neither endorses or opposes any causes. Our primary purpose is to stay sober and help other alcoholics achieve sobriety.

At his very first AA meeting, John met a man named Houston Sewell, a prominent, easygoing, well-liked citizen from the community of nearby Frankfort, Kentucky. He was also a longtime member of Alcoholics Anonymous and the one who started bringing meetings into the narcotics hospital. He believed from his own experience and from working with others that a very large percentage of drug addicts were also alcoholics.

Houston quickly learned that "Dr. 58520" was in complete denial about his alcoholism, which did not surprise him. Little by little, the veteran AA'er helped his new "sponsee" learn about this deadly disease. He encouraged John to share his drinking experiences at the meetings and to talk about the role alcohol played in his life, including the chaos it brought into his family and into his career as a skilled physician.

One evening after the AA meeting concluded, Houston pulled this new member aside and said to him, "I've been listening to you share at our meetings, John. There's something I'd like to say that might help you stop struggling so much with your denial about being an alcoholic. Let's see if we can connect your drinking with your troubles.

"First of all, people we refer to as social drinkers don't drink rubbing alcohol like you did. They don't park their cars in the middle of roads and then wake up in jail charged with public intoxication. They don't check into flophouses and drink quarts of bourbon straight until they're almost dead.

"Social drinkers I know don't get the DT's, that is, unless they really enjoy drinking that awful stuff called paraldehyde. And they may have bad dreams once in a while, but they don't hallucinate. They don't see cockroaches as big as jackrabbits like you did crawling across the curtains and then dropping down into bed with you.

"Also, most skilled surgeons may have a glass of wine with dinner, but not a quart or two of scotch every night when they have to operate the next morning. No, John. From where I sit, you qualify as a class one alcoholic."

That was the night Dr. John Mooney Jr. accepted the fact that he was an alcoholic, that he was totally powerless over booze, that one drink was too many and a thousand not enough, and that he suffered from the threefold disease of alcoholism that affected him physically, mentally, and spiritually.

Houston Sewell told him he might well find the answers to all his problems in the Twelve Steps of AA. Then he handed his "sponsee" what he called "The Big Book of Alcoholics Anonymous" and told him to start reading it and working the program's Twelve Steps to Recovery:

1. We admitted we were powerless over alcohol—that our lives had become unmanageable.
2. Came to believe that a Power greater than ourselves could restore us to sanity.
3. Made a decision to turn our will and our lives over to the care of God as we understood Him.

4. Made a searching and fearless moral inventory of ourselves.

5. Admitted to God, to ourselves, and to another human being the exact nature of our wrongs.

6. Were entirely ready to have God remove all these defects of character.

7. Humbly asked Him to remove our shortcomings.

8. Made a list of all persons we had harmed, and became willing to make amends to them all.

9. Made direct amends to such people wherever possible, except when to do so would injure them or others.

10. Continued to take personal inventory and when we were wrong, promptly admitted it.

11. Sought through prayer and meditation to improve our conscious contact with God as we understood Him, praying only for knowledge of His will and the power to carry that out.

12. Having had a spiritual awakening as the result of these steps, we tried to carry this message to alcoholics, and to practice these principles in all our affairs.

As John began reading the book that was to lead him to a whole new way of life, he was still trying to figure out what his sponsor was all about. "I just couldn't understand Houston Sewell at first," he once explained. "I heard from others in the AA group that he was very rich, drove big automobiles and had houses in Florida and the mountains as well as a beautiful home in Frankfort. Yet here he was sitting around these meetings telling us what a sorry old drunk he was. But he did it with a big smile on his face, like he was a real happy man.

"Houston became my sponsor. He was seventeen years sober at the time and the place he wanted to be the most, despite all that material stuff, was with us drunks, talking about the program and how to get sober and stay sober. This was the most important thing in his life. He was the personification of the AA program and I latched on to it and to him."

One day John was trying to explain to his sponsor how his nervous condition always caused him to get drunk—that if these psychiatrists at the hospital could only solve his nervous condition and straighten out his thinking, then he'd be just fine. Houston grinned and said to him, "So you think your nervous condition gets you drunk. Did you ever think it might be all the whiskey you drank that got you drunk?"

John later remarked, "I never looked at it that way. My nerves didn't get me drunk. The whiskey did. I was on a merry-go-round until Houston set me straight."

Almost five months into his stay at the narcotics hospital, John sat down with Dr. Hawthorne for one of his routine sessions. Only this session was not to be routine. The psychiatrist said the time had come to decide his patient's future course of treatment. He suggested John think about undergoing serious psychoanalysis that might take two or three years to complete.

The startled surgeon explained that he was doing quite well working the AA program and, in all honesty, couldn't see himself staying that long to have his head examined more than it already had been. Then he asked how much longer he would have to remain in the hospital if he didn't accept the recommendation.

"The longest we can keep you here on that court order," Dr. Hawthorne replied, "is about six months for what they call 'the cure.' However, if you decide to stay longer, the U.S. Public Health Service will provide your psychoanalysis treatments free of charge. It's your decision."

While John recognized how much benefit he had received from his stay at Lexington, he hated being locked up. Once again he tried to be as honest with himself as he could be. He believed in his heart that another year or more behind bars might hurt him even more than it would help him. So he turned down the psychiatrist's recommendation.

"Then I strongly suggest," Dr. Hawthorne said, "that you stay in Alcoholics Anonymous and really work the program because there's nowhere else for you to go."

Leaving Dr. Hawthorne's office, John knew the psychiatrist was absolutely right about having nowhere else to go. He had tried so many things before to stay clean and sober and none of them worked. Besides making the rounds of all those dry-out places, he had tried the hobby of woodworking, but the only thing he really made was his neighbors angry for running his loud machine tools late into the night.

He had tried photography but wound up drinking more booze in his darkroom than the amount of fluid he put into his developing pans. He had also bought a T-Bird to make himself feel better. So he realized he should heed Dr. Hawthorne's advice.

As the allotted time for his stay at the hospital began to run out, the now more clear-headed physician found himself suddenly getting very anxious about the thought of going home to Statesboro. He feared facing his family and his friends. As he said later in life, "I got real scared because I felt something bad was going to happen when I left there. I had this crazy man still in my brain who was telling me there wasn't any way in the world I could keep from drinking or drugging once I left.

"I couldn't sleep a wink. I'd lie awake all night worrying. I even told one of the fellows I had gotten close to that I shouldn't leave even if they were going to let me go. But then I learned something I should have known all along—that God works through people.

"My sponsor, Houston, saw what was happening to me. That's when he arranged something with the hospital medical director that hadn't been done in a long time. He was given special permission to take me to an outside meeting of Alcoholics Anonymous. I never will forget it.

"I was allowed to call home first and ask Dot to send me some good clothes right away—my good brown suit along with a shirt, tie, shoes, and a topcoat. Before I hung up, I reminded her of the letter she wrote asking me if I found anything to help me stay sober. I suggested in a very nice way that she hurry out and buy an AA Big Book and read it.

"It was a Tuesday night when Houston picked me up and took me to my first outside meeting of Alcoholics Anonymous at a place in Frankfort called 'The Token Club.' It was my first contact with AA that wasn't in any institution and for a few minutes, I couldn't understand what was going on. The people looked and acted like they were too happy. My first thought was, they're taking something. They're hopped up on something.

"Then I came to realize it wasn't true. This was genuine, just like my sponsor who was always smiling, even when he talked about the worst things that ever happened to him in his life. These were the happiest people I think I have ever seen. I just had to get used to AA humor because it's so different than in the world of social drinkers."

The physician heard someone tell a story that night about blaming others for your problems. He so identified with the story, he would frequently tell it himself later on.

It was about this young lady going to court for a divorce. The judge said, "Suzy, on what grounds do you want this divorce?"

Suzy said, "Judge, I want this divorce on the grounds of infidelity. My husband has been unfaithful to me."

"In what way has your husband been unfaithful to you, Suzy?" the judge asked.

The young lady responded, "Judge, I don't think he's the father of my child."

"I listened to their stories," John continued, "and came to realize they had been down the same road as me. They gave me hope. I knew that somewhere in this program was the answer for me . . . the answer I had been searching for in every dry-out place I had gone to. I felt there was something here that could keep me from getting drunk if I'd stick to it. These people had found it. I made a decision right then that, if I could, I was going to stay with AA people as long as I lived.

"Halfway through the meeting I was asked to say something. My legs shook as I walked to the podium. I simply said I was very grateful to my sponsor for opening my eyes to my disease and that if I followed his suggestions and those in the AA Big Book, I believed I might make it."

After the meeting, a number of people came up to the physician and encouraged him to keep coming back. The last one was a short balding man about his own age. He shook his hand and said, "John, I know you can make it."

It wasn't until the physician got back to the hospital, thanked Houston once again, and headed inside that he suddenly stopped in his tracks and remembered what that balding man at the meeting said to him. He didn't say to the physician that he "might make it." He said, "John, I know you can make it."

It was those words that lessened the fear in the surgeon's gut and enabled him to emerge from Lexington three days later a sober man and a man who now believed he could face whatever the future held—without a drink or a drug.

CHAPTER TWELVE

A Doctor No More

IT WAS AROUND 8 A.M. ON FRIDAY, NOVEMBER 21, 1959, WHEN Houston Sewell picked up his sponsee at the narcotics prison to drive him to the airport in Lexington, Kentucky. He had arranged for John to fly to Atlanta and then connect with another flight that would take him to Savannah where his family would be waiting for him.

There was a chill in the air, and the overcast sky was threatening rain. Houston was chatting away, but the nervous physician wasn't hearing a word. His mind was focused on what was awaiting him and his need to prove he could walk the streets of Statesboro a sober man. And he was trying hard not to listen to the crazy man in his head who was still expressing doubts that it could be done.

John Mooney's AA sponsor walked him to the airport counter and put his arm on his shoulder. He promised to stay in touch and made the physician swear he would attend an AA meeting at home the very next night.

It was a bumpy flight to Atlanta and the plane arrived late. John had to hurry to make his connection.

"When I finally reached the airplane to take me to Savannah," John vividly recalled when sharing his experiences some years later, "I was unable to walk up those steps. Something came over me. It wasn't fear of flying because I loved airplanes. I knew exactly what it was. It was the failure of my pride. I was afraid I might possibly disappoint everybody again and not be able to walk the streets anywhere sober."

He stuck the airplane ticket into his pocket, grabbed a taxi, and headed for downtown Atlanta. He tried not to think about his family waiting at the airport in Savannah.

"I wound up in a hotel room in Atlanta that night, sick and miserable and as helpless as I've ever been in my life. I went into a depression, a deep state of despair. It was absolutely unbearable. I went over to the window and looked down into the street below. I saw the pavement and myself crashing into it headfirst and dying instantly. I remember thinking, 'If this is where it's got to be, then that's it.' I felt I just couldn't go home and face everyone. I think I came closest to jumping out that window that night and destroying myself than I had ever been.

"The depression got worse. I didn't know what to do. Then suddenly I fell to my knees and begged God to help me. I didn't think I had any faith at all left or even any hope that God would do something for me. What I didn't realize was that I had finally reached the point of total surrender. My pride was gone. I was totally destitute of everything. I was powerless and I knew it.

"As I said those words, asking God to help me, the most enormous change came over me, something that had never happened before. Suddenly I felt this tremendous uplift and the sense that everything was going to be all right. The fear went away and I felt a presence of some sort right there with me, carrying me on some kind of a cloud. It has stayed with me my entire life.

"When I think about it even now, it was like what I had been looking for in a bottle—a sense of freedom from everything, that all is right with the world. The problem with alcohol was when I'd almost reach that point, that feeling, I would pass out. Then I'd wake up in a world far worse than the one I had just left.

"Since that night, when I had what I came to realize was a spiritual experience, the need to drink left me. I have never had to fight alcohol since. I haven't had a drink or any type of mood-changing drug or pill since then."

While John was heading for a hotel in Atlanta that day, Dot and their three sons were anxiously waiting at the Savannah airport for his arrival. In fact, in preparation for his return home, Dot had taken her last drink of alcohol earlier that week, on Sunday, November 15. It was the last bottle of cold beer left in the refrigerator. However, she was still taking some pills, which she felt she needed to keep herself steady.

It was her oldest son, Al, who remembered clearly the deep disappointment the whole family experienced when his father never came home that Friday.

"Back at that time," he said, "you could stand behind a chain-link fence as the plane taxied toward you from the runway. We all stood there and watched and waited with a lot of excitement. I believe the plane was a DC-4. It had a nose wheel, a tall upright tail, and the stairway was in the back of the plane.

"I can still see to this day the passengers coming down that stairway. We were all really anxious to see my Daddy appear because he had been gone for so long. But then everyone was off the plane and he wasn't among them. I looked over at my mother. She seemed bewildered, like in a state of shock."

Al said he didn't remember much about the drive back to Statesboro. He only recalls thinking, "Well, yeah. Okay. So my Dad's really dead and this is the way the cowards in my family are telling me this. They just don't have the guts to tell me right out."

John called his wife later that night from Atlanta. He apologized sincerely for missing the plane and disappointing her and the boys. He tried to explain what had happened to him but thought he wasn't making much sense on the telephone. So he promised to be on an early flight the next morning and that he was really looking forward to seeing her.

Dot would later recall that she heard something different in her husband's voice that night. She could tell that the time he had spent in Lexington had changed him more than she realized from all his letters. He said he was close to God now and that it gave him the strength to face all the problems he knew he had created. He assured her they would get through all the debris, that he would work hard again and they would have the wonderful life they always dreamed of having.

While Dot knew she would soon have her husband back sober, those fears that were growing inside her wouldn't go away. The thought of John being sober only increased the terrible feelings she had about herself, the result of her own drinking and drugging. She was frightened that perhaps this man she still loved and always depended upon wouldn't feel the same away about her anymore—that the attraction, the passion, and the desperate need they once had for each other would fade away as their new sober lives together began. It was a foreboding that stayed with her for some time.

On the way home from the airport the next day, her son Jimmy remembered the strange impression his father made on him as he spoke in a happy and upbeat manner with his family.

"There was such an obvious change in my dad that I couldn't help but notice it," he said. "It seemed like he went away somewhere one kind of person and now came back a different kind of person. It was the same body, but there was a different man in it."

Young Bobby only recalled how much his dad kept hugging him and promised he would never leave them again for such a long time. He also remembered the happy look on his mother's face that whole day.

But again, it was John's oldest son, Al, who never forgot what happened later that night.

"Dad came upstairs as we were all getting ready to go to bed. He had us all climb onto my bed and said he needed to talk to us about something. I don't remember all the details of what he said, except that it was the first believable conversation I've ever had with my dad in my whole life.

"He told us he had been in prison. Immediately the pieces in my head all came together. He said he had been in a lot of trouble, that he had done things and been places that he would never have chosen to be in had he been in his right mind.

"But he said he learned he had a disease called alcoholism that caused him to do those things. While he was away, he said he met some people like himself who had found the answer to his problem. Then he started talking about AA, and I was clueless. I thought AA was like the army paratroopers or something—soldiers helping other soldiers.

"He said he had a spiritual experience, something he couldn't really explain, but something that made a big difference in his life. He said he was now much closer to God and went on to talk about spiritual stuff, not about the church we went to or the Bible, but how much God loves us all.

"Then he reached out and poked each of us—Jimmy, Bobby, and myself—in the chest near our hearts with his finger. He said, 'There's a little bit of God in all three of you.' Then he pointed downstairs and said, 'And in your mother, too.'

"And then he knelt down and said some prayers with us. It was an experience with my dad that I will never forget. I came to realize later on that it was his way of beginning to make amends to us for not being the father he had always wanted to be."

The newly inspired physician didn't make an AA meeting that night or the next, as his sponsor had strongly suggested. Instead he went to bed thinking about all he had to do being home, including rebuilding his loving relationship with the woman now cuddled warmly in his arms.

Yes, John certainly remembered Houston Sewell's telling him he went to five, six, sometimes seven meetings a week. But then, this dedicated man was retired. He could do all that. Maybe, John thought, someday I'll be able to do that too, but right now I have to get back to being a busy doctor. I have to rebuild my practice, support my family, pay my debts. I will definitely try to make at least one AA meeting every month. He actually went to sleep that night feeling he had just made a rather generous commitment to the program that helped him find the solution to his problems.

The physician was in his office the first thing Monday morning when his good friend Dr. Jack Averitt dropped by. The professor was both surprised and pleased by what he saw. He wrote later in his journal: "John looked well, his attitude was positive, he had gained some weight and his complexion was ruddy and healthy looking. His usual extravert manner was somewhat subdued and I interpreted this as an outward manifestation of an inward humility which I thought was great. So I wasn't surprised that within a matter of days, his waiting room was filled with patients anxious to see him."

The physician had another friend visit the following day. It was Henry, the man who tried making a "Twelve-Step call" at his house sometime ago, hoping to take him to an AA meeting. Henry had heard through the grapevine that Dr. Mooney had joined the fellowship in prison and he was looking forward to going to meetings with the good doctor on a regular basis.

But the avid AA member struck out once again, only this time it wasn't because the newly sober physician wanted to drink. It was because the newly sober physician felt he was too busy to do something that might keep the chaos out of his life. However, he did tell Henry he would probably see him at a meeting in a few weeks, if time permitted.

Perhaps John thought that his experience in the hotel room in Atlanta was all he needed to stay sober—that turning his life over to God's care would provide him with all the strength and insight he needed. He was about to learn that his God worked in wonderful and mysterious ways for people who love Him—often in ways that we don't understand at first.

Dallas Cason was naturally delighted to have Dr. Mooney back. She couldn't get over the big change that had taken place, and John couldn't thank her enough for all she had done to hold things together while he was gone. And with so many patients, both old and new, coming for treatment, it seemed like old times—"even better than old times," the nurse quipped.

Then on Thursday afternoon, December 4, a special delivery letter arrived from the Georgia Composite Medical Board in Atlanta. Dallas took it in to her boss and watched his face turn white as he read it. John often shared that frightful moment when he would speak at AA meetings.

"The Medical Board said, 'Dr. Mooney, you have been convicted of a felony. You cannot practice medicine in the State of Georgia with a felony conviction on your record.' So they revoked my license and ordered me to appear at a hearing in Atlanta the very next day.

"It floored me. I remember thinking, I did everything they told me to do up there at that narcotics prison and now this has to happen. Then, for some strange reason which I now know was my Higher Power talking to me, I remembered something my sponsor, Houston Sewell, once told me.

"He said when bad things happen, just wait and be patient. We never know what God has planned for us. So I didn't drink. Instead, I called my good friend Dr. Jack Averitt and sought his counsel."

The professor recalled that it was around 4:30 in the afternoon when he received an urgent call from his good friend, whose voice was filled with anxiety. He said simply, "Jack, I need your help. Is it possible you can come to my office right away?"

Jack had just arrived home from Georgia Southern, so he went immediately. John showed him the letter revoking his license and the demand that he appear at a hearing in Atlanta the following day. The professor recalled John saying to him, "You have already helped me so much, Jack. You have given me your time, your guidance and your energy, things that money cannot pay for. That's why I'm reluctant to ask, but I would like you to come to this hearing with Dot and me if you possibly can."

Dr. Averitt read the letter again. He thought, had not this man already gone through enough at this point? This has to be the last straw. I can't let him down now.

So once again the professor managed to find a substitute to handle his classes at the university, and at five o'clock that Friday morning, December 5, he, Dot, and John were on their way to Atlanta.

"We parked in the lot across from the capitol," Jack later wrote in his journal. "We entered the building twenty minutes before the appointed hour of nine o'clock. A receptionist directed us to the meeting room. We watched the committee members—all physicians—enter one by one. Dot was so nervous she had tears in her eyes.

"The committee chairman asked each of us to identify ourselves. He then said only the doctor charged with an offense could remain in the committee room during the hearing. I politely explained I was one of Dr. Mooney's closest friends and asked if I could make a brief statement before leaving. The answer was in the affirmative.

"I confirmed my intimate knowledge of John's problem through the past years and how his problem had become more acute and advanced in the past two years. I also described briefly my involvement in his rehabilitation process, emphasizing that the Lord had directed me in this endeavor and that my faith was strong enough to believe that Dr. Mooney could find a solution to his problem which he has.

"Since I was not a physician or an attorney, I cited my professional credentials and my record of fifteen years of leadership as a dean at Georgia Southern. I was then interrupted by a question from the committee chairman.

"He asked if I believed that the responsibility of the Medical Board in licensing physicians should not be monitored with such care that patients and potential patients would be protected from any mistakes, incorrect decisions or injuries that could occur when one is not in control of his or her faculties.

"I replied that I totally agreed and that the physician who was appearing before the committee had failed to meet some of those obligations during his past practice of medicine. I insisted that I did not subscribe to the philosophy that because he was not the only one who violated the standards of his profession that he should be excused.

"I added, however, that this man had undergone a strenuous period of rehabilitation and treatment. According to the authorities dealing with the problem, he was released from the institution to which he had been committed for six months, cured of his problem and able to return to the practice of medicine.

"Then I went on to say that if Dr. Mooney's license is revoked permanently, I would take it as a personal challenge to stump the entire state of Georgia to make sure that no physician licensed by this Medical Board shall be permitted to practice medicine if he has ever been under the influence of alcohol while treating a patient in his office or performing duties in a hospital.

"I asked the committee chairman and the other members of the Board not to take my statement as a threat. I said I was merely informing them that I would become the personal leader of a crusade that would make sure the regulations imposed on Dr. Mooney would apply universally to all physicians. I might fail in that task, I added, but I would bring the medical profession into such focus with the people of Georgia that the crusade would not end there.

"I then thanked the committee for listening to my remarks. I concluded by expressing my belief that the proper and legitimate decision would come from the esteemed committee in order to assist a man who was highly trained to minister to the physical problems of others and who had already suffered enough on his road to recovery."

After testifying for more than an hour, John was told the Medical Board would make a decision by noon. So he, Dot, and Dr. Averitt sat outside in the hallway to await the news.

The Medical Board decided to suspend the physician's license for a period of six months. It was made clear that if he continued in his manner of adjustment and led a well-disciplined life, he could return for another hearing before the board and potentially be allowed to return to private practice as a licensed physician.

On the drive back to Statesboro, John tried to calm his wife's concerns about sustaining their family and paying their bills during the months ahead. Although he would have to close his practice for the time being, he believed he could find other ways to bring in some income. His friend Jack suggested that perhaps the Medical Board considered their decision to be in the same light as a patient convalescing following surgery—that they felt John needed more time to completely recover.

By the time they arrived home, the sober physician knew exactly why the board members made the decision they did.

"God had them take my license away so I could get my sanity back," he would often say at AA meetings. "I thought I knew everything about the recovery program, but I didn't know the least bit. I had never really gotten into the Twelve Steps of Recovery. Yes, I had a spiritual experience and felt close to God, but my thinking was still all screwed up—like only needing to go to a meeting once a month. Now God was giving me the time to really get well.

"Because it was still all about me. I had to get back to being a busy doctor right away. My patients needed me and I needed the money. I had to repay all my debts right away so my friends would think well of me. I had to be a big success so my wife and children would be proud of me. That night I got down on my knees and did what Houston Sewell used to tell me to do at the prison—turn my will and my life over to the care of God."

The next morning John sat down with Dallas Cason and explained the situation. She understood completely and told him she was confident he would be back in business in six months. She said she could pick up various nursing assignments in the meantime. She also offered to help him put out a notice to all his patients, explaining that he could consult with them on medical matters but would not be able to treat them for a while.

That afternoon before he closed his office, John picked up the telephone and called his old friend Henry. He said he wouldn't be busy for the next several months and would like to get involved with AA. Henry was absolutely delighted. He picked up the physician that night and took him to his first AA meeting in Statesboro. Dot came along to support her husband.

"I was very nervous, seeing some people I had known over the years," the surgeon would recall, "especially when they asked me to say a few words. I spoke for about ten minutes, telling them about the rehabilitation program I had been through in Lexington. Everyone seemed so serious that I decided to tell a funny story my father used to tell just to loosen things up. I said the story explained how screwed up I still was.

"This guy was overseas during World War II and wrote his father a letter saying, 'Daddy, I can't tell you where I am, but I shot a polar bear yesterday.' Then a few months later, he got another letter saying, 'Daddy, I can't tell you where I am, but I've been transferred. However, yesterday I danced with a hula girl.' And then a little later, the father got another letter. It said, 'Daddy, I can't tell you where I am, except I'm in a hospital. I should have shot the hula girl and danced with the polar bear.'

"A few people laughed, maybe trying to be polite. But when the meeting ended, two other people I had known before came over to speak with Dot and me. One was C. D., who had a big cigar in his mouth, and the other was his wife, Ida, who wore a funny little hat. They both said it was the worst AA talk ever made in the state of Georgia and burst out laughing. Then C. D. invited us back to their house for some coffee and cake.

"He and Ida played us tapes of some really good AA talks. We then discussed them and spoke about the AA program into the wee hours of the morning. They said they would pick us up the next night at six o'clock, and they did. We went to Walterboro for a meeting and the following night to Macon. Then we went to Augusta and Savannah and somewhere every night. We were going, going, going. And because I had the time and little else to do, I threw myself totally into Alcoholics Anonymous and Dot came along for the ride."

Although Dot Mooney willingly accompanied her husband to all these meetings, she kept telling herself she was only doing it to support the wonderful effort he was making to stay sober. She was still in denial that she was an alcoholic. In fact, she would attend Al-Anon meetings, a support group for the families and friends of alcoholics, if there was one in the town to which they were going.

"But I would make sure that everybody knew John was the alcoholic and that I was going to Al-Anon," she often said with a laugh. "And I really did love Al-Anon and could identify with almost everything that was said in meetings. However, as I listened more and more at open AA meetings, I started identifying more with the alcoholics.

"I was really conflicted until one night when I heard this AA old-timer named Virgil. Old-timers have a habit of saying the damnedest things. Virgil said, 'If you're sitting back there taking pills, you would be better off drinking your liquor.'

"I hadn't had a drink of whiskey or beer since the week before my husband came home. I didn't want to tempt him by having him smell it on my breath. But I was still taking pills—one before meals, one after meals, between meals, at bedtime, even sometimes during an AA meeting. They seemed to lessen my desire to drink. When that old-timer said that, something clicked.

"I went home and threw all my pills away. I flushed them down the toilet. I didn't know much about this withdrawal stuff or convulsions. I only knew those things could happen if you took hard drugs. I didn't realize I could have died. But from that point on, I got real serious about the AA program."

At the same time, John was beginning to get bored with AA and all the running around. He was still relying on Houston Sewell as a sponsor instead of finding someone in or around Statesboro he could see and talk with more often. He was having difficulty understanding and working some of the program's Twelve Steps.

"One morning I was downtown sitting at the counter in one of our local drugstores having a cup of coffee with this friend of mine, Joe," the physician shared at an AA meeting. "We had joined the program in Statesboro about the same time. He was talking about C. D. and Ida, that they were fanatics about going to so many meetings. Joe said there's such a thing as getting too much of AA, getting so fanatical that you don't have anything else in your life.

"I was nodding along with him, especially when he said AA was running out of his ears. I felt it was running out of my ears too. So that night I stretched out on the parlor couch and said to Dot, 'Honey, I haven't seen *Gunsmoke* in three months. And I haven't kept up with the news. I've been making so many meetings I think AA is getting under my skin. So I'm going to stay home tonight and watch television.'

"Dot was putting on her earrings but she never missed a lick. She said I could just lie there and watch television if I wanted to, but she was going with C. D. and Ida to the AA meeting in Dublin. Then she remarked that she didn't want to take the chance of missing the one meeting that might keep her sober. So I got up like a little puppy dog and went with her.

"A few nights later, somebody came up to me at a meeting and asked if I had heard about my friend, Joe. He got drunk. Here was the guy I was agreeing with about being too fanatical when it came to AA. I learned that when you begin to find fault with the AA program, there's usually something wrong with you. That's also when I got a sponsor closer to home named Corneil Foy and began working with him on the Twelve Steps. Today I wear the program like a comfortable-fitting suit. It's never been boring since."

While Dot was also trying her best to practice the Twelve Steps of AA in her life, she was having difficulty with her low self-esteem—the bad feelings she still had about herself that translated into a fear of John not loving her the way he used to. Also, she felt her husband was spending so much time with his new AA friends and trying to help newcomers that he was spending less time with her. Without realizing it at first, it was beginning to spark a touch of jealousy that led to a growing resentment. "For some reason," she once said, "I got all mixed up. John seemed to be making more progress in the program than I was. I even began to resent him for sleeping so soundly because he seemed to have so much peace and contentment in his life. I didn't feel part of that. In fact, I thought he didn't need me like he used to, so I decided I didn't need him either.

"One night he snored one too many times. For some reason I lost it and started pounding on him. In fact, I tried to knock the holy hell out of him. He sat up with a start and said, 'What do you want?' I shouted, 'I want a divorce!'

"His eyes opened wide and I'll never forget the shocked look on his face. He asked, 'What the hell for?' I yelled, 'Because you sleep like you do and snore too much! No, because you don't love me! You have never loved me! You don't love the children! And there's something you need to know. I don't love you either! I have never loved you!'

"Now, here I was shouting at a man who's sober, a pretty smart man who has a wonderful program to live by. And he's living it. He doesn't get upset. He doesn't get angry. Instead, he moves very close to me and says, 'Well, I'll tell you one thing, my dear. I love you more than anybody I've ever loved in my life. I'm happier now than I've ever been in my life. I can't stop you if a divorce is what you want, but I'll have no part of it.' Then he kissed me on the cheek, laid back down, and went to sleep.

"And would you believe it. After all that, I wiped the tears from my eyes, laid back down, and also went right to sleep. You see, this was my insecurity talking, my fear and my anxiety. I thought he was just too much of a gentleman to leave me when I was so sick. But now I knew that John really loved me and always had. That's all I needed to know. I've never had a problem about his feelings for me ever since."

Less than two months later, in March of 1960 and at the age of thirty-seven, Dot Mooney found herself pregnant with her fourth child. She and John were ecstatic. While some of those old fears concerning her drinking and drugging came back, she now had a Twelve-Step program and a strong relationship with her God to handle them.

John had other things to handle. Although AA was now the first and most important thing in his life and always would be, he had to figure out how to resolve his mounting debt problems, his serious tax situation with the IRS, and ways to find some income to provide for his family.

So he turned once again to his good friend Earl Dabbs. Since the young accountant had spent several years working for the Internal Revenue Service, he arranged a meeting at his office with the two IRS agents working on the physician's case. Having John present, and with his permission, Earl openly detailed the circumstances of the back-tax problem and what caused it. He was completely honest with the agents, explaining there was no income at the present time since the Medical Board had revoked the surgeon's license.

It was agreed that John would begin paying his regular taxes just as soon as he was able to practice medicine again. He also agreed to a delayed payment plan for his back taxes. In addition, Earl persuaded the agents to lower the amount owed and not to charge any more interest and penalties. The physician expressed his gratitude to the sharp accountant for all his help, which only strengthened their relationship even more.

Then John went to those around town to whom he owed money, apologizing for taking advantage of their friendship. He promised to repay them whenever he was able to reopen his medical practice, hopefully in a matter of months. He also wrote to other creditors, expressing the same sentiments. His openness and honesty were generally well received. In most cases, people were simply glad to have him back in Statesboro—healthy and sober.

"I found out that people were more interested in the man than they were in the actual money," he once explained. "If the man's all right, the money is going to be okay. I discovered that every account I owed gave me a chance. For example, we had a fairly new station wagon that I had financed but could no longer make payments on. So I was going to turn it back to the dealer. There was no way I could keep it, at least honestly.

"The owner of the dealership asked me if I needed the car. I told him that I sure did but wasn't in a position to keep up the payments. We went into his office and he called General Motors Acceptance Corporation, which financed the car. The owner vouched for me. They told him they would suspend the payments for six months if I was sure I could start paying at that point. I said I thought so, but wasn't absolutely sure. They said to let me keep the car anyway and trust I'd do my best. That's what happens when you try to be honest with yourself and others."

A short time later, the surgeon ran into another old friend, Leodel Coleman, the editor of the *Bulloch Herald*. They met at a meeting of the Rotary Club, an organization John had been a member of for many years. The editor was quite impressed by "the new Dr. Mooney," and also by his interest in current events and their effects on the people in town.

A few days later, Leodel Coleman called and asked the doctor to drop by his office. He wondered if he would have any interest in writing a daily column for the newspaper. Of course, he would be paid and could choose whatever subjects he cared to expound upon. It didn't take very long for them to cut a deal.

John was thrilled. So was Dot, especially over the prospect of having some income to count on. After returning from their AA meeting that evening, they stayed up late discussing ideas and subjects John might write about.

John's first column appeared in the *Bulloch Herald* on January 21, 1960. It was titled "Never Take Yourself Too Seriously." The subject he had chosen was the controversy raging at that time in the state of Georgia over school integration. Some excerpts from the column read:

"When confronted with problems like integration and the variety of opinions and intense feelings which accompany such discussions, one wonders why persons born, reared and educated in the same area, in this case The South, should offer such extreme solutions without considering the realistic rather than the unrealistic affect on the community.

"Some predict there might be a mass exodus of people from the state of Georgia. Industry might leave us. New industry might shun us. And when the time came to reopen the schools, that is, if it were decided to do so, the teachers might be employed somewhere else. And our college students, out of the family and on their own, might be enrolled in far off colleges and universities.

"The possible effects on our economy are fantastic, even calamitous, our educators warn. But are these predictions truly realistic, or could we be taking our prejudices just a little too seriously."

While the surgeon felt challenged at times to cover current events, he preferred to write mostly about people's health needs, getting regular physical checkups, civic projects like blood drives, and emotional problems like the effects of fear and anxiety on one's life. For example, he did a series of columns about anxiety, one of them titled "Anxiety Is the Failure to Accept Life as It Really Is." Among the points John Mooney made were these:

"Anxiety always seems to concern something which is not happening to us at the moment. Since the multitude of events which are not happening to us range from the possible breaking of a shoe string in a little while to the apocalyptic disintegration of the Universe before I finish writing this column, you can see that the sources of anxiety are unlimited.

"It appears that anxiety can be classified, practically, in only one way, by time. Using this method, anxiety can exist: 1, concerning things which have or have not happened to us in the past; 2, concerning things which will or will not happen to us in the future; 3, concerning things which are not happening to us right now. All of these we can do nothing about, so why be anxious about them?

"Do we need tranquilizers for our anxiety or mood-altering drugs? Or is anxiety perhaps a lack of faith or a denial of God. If it is, then the conflict going on within an anxious person could be more vital than appears on the surface. To relieve the agony of such a struggle between mind, body and soul, people feel they might need all the tranquilizers, narcotics, sedatives and alcohol they can get.

"So, take heart pharmaceutical manufacturers. With limitless horizons for worry and anxiety, we can swallow all the soothing drugs you can produce. But don't make any financial donations to churches or religious organizations because God could put you out of business."

In another column on anxiety the doctor wrote:

"Seeing anxiety as a major obstacle on the road to happiness, we can begin to tear it apart and throw it into the ditch a little bit at a time. Let's start by living 24 hours today, leaving yesterday to the past where it has gone and is not recoverable, and making flexible plans for tomorrow.

"Since anxiety can vanish when we improve our relationship

with God, we should think of praying. Here is a tried and true prayer which can lead a straight and sure path through the most harassing anxiety.

"God grant me the Serenity to accept the things I cannot change, Courage to change the things I can and Wisdom to know the difference."

Naturally, the newborn sober journalist also found time to write a number of columns about Alcoholics Anonymous, what it is and how it offers a solution to those in desperate straits from drinking. In a column titled "AA Helps Those Who Come Seeking Help," he wrote:

"Alcoholism is recognized by the medical profession as an incurable disease. Once a person has become an alcoholic, he can never be a social drinker again. Efforts by physicians and psychiatrists as well as ministers and social and religious organizations to help the alcoholic stop drinking are generally ineffective. They have a recovery rate of about one or two percent.

"In AA, the recovery rate is 75 percent. About half of those who enter Alcoholics Anonymous with an honest desire to stop drinking stay sober permanently. Another 25 percent sober up after one or more relapses. Theoretically, the AA program should be 100 percent effective. However, the remaining 25 percent fail to stay sober usually because of mental disease, brain damage from drinking or a constitutional inability to be honest with themselves."

To keep the Georgia Medical Board in Atlanta apprised of his progress, the physician sent his columns to each committee member along with a report on his activities in AA. Dr. Averitt also wrote the board monthly, commenting on his good friend's reintegration into the Statesboro community and the integrity of his sobriety. And on occasion, a board representative would visit Statesboro for a chat with the physician.

Almost six months to the day his medical license had been suspended, Dr. John Mooney Jr. received word that he would be permitted to resume his medical practice. Dot wept in his arms as he felt their baby kick in her belly. That night he went to his regular AA meeting and told the group about another miracle that had just happened in his life because of staying sober in the program and following the Will of his Higher Power. He also informed them he would be open for business in a week.

One of the first people he called to tell about the good news was his friend Jack.

"He had so much joy in his voice," the professor later wrote. "I was also happy for him, not just because he had his medical license back, but also because I was overdue for a physical check-up and I wanted to see my doctor again.

"On my initial visit, Dallas informed me that John told her not to charge me for my visits. This I refused to accept. I walked back to his office and explained to him that my actions could not be bought and paid for. They were voluntary. I came to see him for professional services and I intended to pay for it. If I ever felt the fee was excessive, I would question it. John simply smiled and shook his head."

The next miracle that happened in the lives of John and Dot Mooney occurred on October 20, 1960. That's the day Dot gave birth to a beautiful baby girl. She named her Carol Lind Mooney.

CHAPTER THIRTEEN

The Crazy House on Lee Street

IT WAS 1960. IT WAS A LEAP YEAR AND A PERIOD THAT WAS TO be filled with historical significance.

It was the year that marked the start of the "sexual revolution." Hugh Hefner opened the first Playboy Club in Chicago. Chubby Checker exploded onto the scene with "The Twist." Elvis Presley returned home from the service and quickly hit the top of the charts with "It's Now or Never" and "Are You Lonesome Tonight?"

The laser and the heart pacemaker were invented. The first American troops were sent to Vietnam. The Supreme Court declared segregation in interstate public transportation illegal. A United Airlines DC-8 collided in midair with a TWA Lockheed Constellation over New York City, killing more than two hundred people.

The Soviets shot down an American U-2 spy plane and sentenced pilot Gary Powers to ten years in prison for espionage. As the Cold War heated up, Soviet Premier Nikita Khrushchev pounded his shoe at the United Nations General Assembly and threatened to annihilate all of Europe.

Pete Rozelle became commissioner of the National Football League. Jack Paar quit TV for the first time. Cassius Clay (who later changed his name to Muhammad Ali) won the Light Heavyweight gold medal for boxing at the Summer Olympic Games, and the U.S. hockey team won a gold medal at the Winter Olympic Games. *Ben-Hur* and Charlton Heston won Academy Awards.

But the biggest event of 1960 was the election of John F. Kennedy, the youngest U.S. president in the nation's history, and Americans across the country suddenly felt less fearful and more hopeful for a bright new future.

And so did John and Dot Mooney in Statesboro, Georgia.

Like Dr. Mooney, President Kennedy was also a war hero, having won the Navy Cross and a Purple Heart for his actions commanding a PT boat in the South Pacific. And as a result of his election, the entire country, including the Mooneys, believed they were on the verge of a rebirth of the spirit, especially after the president challenged them in his first inaugural address: "Ask not what your country can do for you, ask what you can do for your country."

Yes, it was a time of great promise, great anticipation, and great dreams. The physician and his wife could sense it. In spite of all they had been through, they no longer saw dark clouds on the horizon. They saw a bright new dream, and this youthful and encouraging new president symbolized it for them and for the nation.

However, like JFK, who had much to do to achieve his promised goals, so did Dr. Mooney. And now with his license back to practice medicine, he was ready to roll up his sleeves and get to work.

The physician was convinced that the will of his Higher Power was for him to build an even more successful and more lucrative practice than he had before and to use his surgical skills to become the most sought-after surgeon in the South. This would put him in a position to clean up his debts quickly, and all the other problems in his life as well. But as he once shared with some AA friends, "I still had no idea what doing God's will really meant. I was going along thinking that because these things that I wanted to do were good, that they were helpful to people, God was going to approve of them. I had no idea I was doing my will, not His, until I found myself being pulled in another direction.

"I discovered that I didn't really know what God wanted from me. I learned I had to pray and ask Him. Now I do that every single morning. I ask, 'God, please show me the way. Show me what it is you want me to do today.'

"I let my Higher Power guide me now, lead me because I don't know. I can't be sure from one minute to the next. He may change His plans for me and find something else as He often does. I have to keep alert to this all the time."

What began pulling the physician in another direction was the growing awareness among his medical colleagues, not just in Statesboro but elsewhere, that he knew from personal experience how to help alcoholics. And the longer he was sober, and the more he spoke at meetings throughout the Southeast, the more that word spread.

Even before John had gotten his medical license back, some doctors were asking him to help them counsel their alcoholic patients, including women.

"That's when I'd have to ask Dot for her help," he'd quip, "particularly after she had sworn off anything stronger than a cup of decaffeinated coffee."

Although the physician and his wife didn't know it at the time, this was the beginning of a whole new direction in their lives. It was a direction their Higher Power had apparently chosen for them, and once they recognized it, they both fully embraced it.

"By the end of that first year after my license was reinstated," John recalled, "more and more alcoholic patients began appearing at my office. Some of them were sicker than others. Many of them needed more than counseling or an AA meeting. They required detoxing and medical attention.

"I came to realize that there are some people who are just too sick to get well right away by simply attending AA meetings. Alcoholism can do great physical and mental damage. These are the people who come to AA for a short time and leave. They come back and leave again because they are so sick mentally, physically, and spiritually. Most of them require special treatment— time to get their bodies physically better and their brains cleaned out of all the substances they have been taking. So at first, I outfitted two rooms in my office as bedrooms to treat those in the worse shape."

His nurse, Dallas, was happy to be back with her boss and working with him to handle his old and new patients, as well as the growing number of alcoholics. The thing that impressed her the most was John's total dedication to Alcoholics Anonymous.

"We could have an office filled with patients," she said, "and Dr. Mooney would get a call about an alcoholic badly in need of his services. He'd drop everything, including his patients, and leave. It bothered me at first until one day he explained that it was AA that kept him sober, and without being sober, he wouldn't have anything, especially an office filled with patients."

Before and after Dot's pregnancy, she and her husband shared their recovery stories in many places. In addition to speaking at AA gatherings, they were also invited to share their experience with addiction at some medical and scientific conferences and small psychiatric forums. As a result, many alcoholic patients were being recommended to John from out of state, including a growing number of impaired physicians.

"If they arrived intoxicated, which was usually the case," the physician said, "I admitted them to Bulloch County Hospital right down the road for detox. Less serious cases I put into the rooms at my office or into rooms at the nearby Norris Hotel. As they began to feel better, I would take them to AA meetings."

The system he set up worked pretty well for several years. Eventually, however, a committee of John's colleagues from the hospital told him the increasing volume of out-of-state alcoholics was making it difficult for them to find private rooms in the hospital for their own patients. Henceforth, only alcoholics from Statesboro and five surrounding counties could be admitted. They said local needs had to come first, and the only exceptions would be extremely ill patients who required hospital care—provided a basic detoxification unit were set up somewhere else, for example, at John's office.

Even though the physician was now caring for a growing number of alcohol and drug abusers, his hard work and dedication helped his medical practice prosper. Former patients returned. New ones came, and the need for his surgical skills kept him constantly busy. Still, he never neglected his AA meetings or his AA commitments.

And he put his newfound prosperity to good use. In less than three years, John had paid off all his creditors, including the IRS, and was earning enough to meet Dot's heartfelt request. She wanted to remodel their Lee Street home to give each of their four children their own room. Also, she had been watching the rapid rise in her husband's addicted clientele and the problems he was having about where to treat the sickest ones. Her intuition suggested they add a couple of guest rooms to their expansion plans. John could afford it, so they did. They rented a house nearby until the remodeling was done.

In November 1966, a seriously impaired doctor from Atlanta staggered into town. He had heard about Dr. Mooney and his intimate knowledge of alcoholism and came to be treated. The man was on the verge of the DTs, but there was no detox space available anywhere. John took him home that night and put him in one of the guest bedrooms, where he detoxed him. The very next day, after discussing it with Dot, the surgeon went to Statesboro's city hall seeking official approval to operate their Lee Street home as a boardinghouse. He received permission without a problem.

That was the beginning. From that point on, the number of alcoholic and drug-addicted patients continued to increase. Dot once explained, "When we ran out of guest bedrooms, we moved the furniture out of the dining room and replaced it with five beds. It became the place where we detoxed all the new arrivals instead of at John's office. I had a large, beautiful chandelier hanging in the center of the dining room ceiling. It was often the first object a patient saw coming out from under the influence of alcohol. Some thought they had died and gone to Heaven. The room became known as the Chandelier Room. We also had a floor-to-ceiling mirror on one wall. I'd see people get up, look into the mirror, and say, 'Hello. How are you today?' They didn't realize they were talking to themselves. I'd laugh because I used to do the same thing when I was in my cups.

"Our oldest boys, Al and Jimmy, left for college, so their rooms went next. Our son Bobby, who was fifteen, moved into a small log cabin we had built in the backyard. For Carol Lind, who had just turned seven, we installed a partition in the living room right next to what had become the nursing station. But it was roomy and she had a nice, comfortable twin bed to sleep in.

"John and I slept in our own bedroom downstairs, away from most of the commotion. However, occasionally we'd get a knock on the front door from someone who had been drinking rather heavily and was looking for help to stop. We'd set up a cot in the living room, which was right across from our bedroom, and watch them until they went to sleep. The next day if they were up to it, we'd take them to an AA meeting along with others who were living in the house and getting well.

"Anyway, that's how we started. The AA Big Book told John and me that one of the best ways to stay sober was to get busy helping newcomers and others who were having serious problems making the program. We were finding such a wonderful life in sobriety that we didn't want to lose it—and we wanted even more. So we followed the Big Book's advice and counseled everyone who came through Lee Street the same way—according to the program laid out in the Big Book."

More than fifty years ago, most people knew little about alcoholism. The American Medical Association hadn't declared alcoholism an incurable disease until 1956. Also, as John and Dot Mooney would often point out, back then there were very few places one could take a seriously ill alcoholic who couldn't afford one of the few addiction treatment centers around the country. In Georgia, for example, most destitute alcoholics were sent to the state insane asylum in Milledgeville. Its motto was said to be "Many went in but few came out."

"Patients came from as far away as New York, Texas, Ohio, Florida, and Michigan," Dot remembered. "At one point, we had three men at the house who had just left prison and were struggling to stay sober. They were all in one room. We had three drunken women from fleabag hotels who were now on rollaway beds in our living room. And all the guest bedrooms were filled with other very sick alcoholics. At one point we had twenty-six people, including five family members, living at the house all at the same time.

"This illness is cunning, baffling, and powerful. That's why we got into it full force."

The simple goal that John and Dot Mooney set for all those treated at their home was to get them well enough physically and mentally so they could live a sober life on their own through the spiritual program of Alcoholics Anonymous.

To an objective observer, life at Lee Street was far from boring. One might say it could seem frantic at times, perhaps eerie or scary at other times, but certainly hopeful, uplifting, and loving most of the time. Some alcoholics might stay there a few days, others a few weeks or a few months, and others maybe a year. Some former patients who went through the house and are still sober fondly remember the place as "the crazy house on Lee Street." When a wino would be detoxing under the chandelier in the dining room and a frightened woman convulsing on the kitchen floor, one could well understand the "crazy house" designation.

For the Mooney children still living at home, the abnormal once again seemed almost normal.

"I remember there was always a lot of laughing in the house," Jimmy Mooney recalled. "Sure, once in a while you'd notice someone pretty sick, but most of the time everybody seemed to be smiling, at least when they were talking to me or one of my brothers or my sister. And everything revolved around Alcoholics Anonymous. I didn't understand it at first, but then my folks got me involved in Alateen and I started to learn a lot more about the program. I was probably twelve at the time."

Alateen, like Al-Anon, is a Twelve-Step program designed to help the children of alcoholics recover from the effects the disease has on them and their families.

"Mom and Dad would carry us kids to AA meetings with them all over the place," the middle son explained. "Later on, when my dad started speaking at AA conventions out of town, they would load us all up and take us there too. What I enjoyed most is there would be a special room for Alateen members. It was like our own hospitality room. We had lots of food and soda and music and stuff for us kids to do. To be perfectly honest, I don't think I went to Alateen to try and get better or to get help for myself. It was just there was a real attractiveness there, something special about the people and even the kids who were trying to work the program. I looked up to them."

While Jimmy's older brother, Al, also attended Alateen and even started an Alateen group in Statesboro, it didn't do much to relieve him of some angry feelings he had built up against his father during his growing-up years. He honestly admitted they got even worse after his father found sobriety.

"I felt that Alcoholics Anonymous had stolen my father from me," he said rather bluntly, "and I resented it. I hadn't done much with my father for years and years. And now he comes home from prison sober, and instead of spending time with me or any of us, he's working all day and going to AA meetings practically every night of the week.

"His AA friends would babysit us. Then as I got older, I would babysit Jimmy and Bobby and Carol Lind when she came along. Sometimes my dad and my mother would take all of us to AA meetings with them. But I still never spent any time with my dad. He was always with AA people. I went from once thinking he was dead to now wondering why he didn't want anything to do with me. It was a difficult period I went through.

"Of course I didn't realize or appreciate at the time what AA was all about and why my father needed it so much. I'm very grateful we were able to resolve our differences later on."

As for life at Lee Street, the Mooneys' oldest son has few vivid recollections of the day-to-day events there. By the time the house became filled with recovering alcoholics, he had left for Emory University in Atlanta to study pre-med and follow in his father's footsteps. Jimmy would also leave soon after for Georgia Southwestern College. On the other hand, their younger brother, Bobby, did recall quite a few things about this rather "unusual" period in his growing-up years.

"It was an insane environment even before my parents started bringing alcoholics into our house," Bobby smiled. "I mean, if you step back and take a look at the whole picture, it was crazy. You know, my mother was barely sober, maybe a few years. She had three boys she had raised while she was using alcohol and drugs, and now she also had a little baby girl. She probably looked around and said, 'Where the hell did they all come from?'

"And we boys were hellions. Excuse me. Not my brother Al. He was the perfect kid and I resented the hell out of him. But me and Jimmy were rotten to the core."

Being the youngest son, he said his mother tried very hard to be loving and affectionate most of the time, especially since she was now sober. But there were times when either he or Jimmy would do something that would cause her to go off—"to become real mean and angry." Bobby, who also went on to became a doctor like his father, recalled one incident in particular.

"I'll never forget one of the worst whippings I ever got," he said. "I was babysitting Carol Lind and really messed up. Carol Lind was about three and I was around nine. Mama had gone off somewhere and warned me to keep a close eye on her.

"Jimmy and some of his friends were playing outside the house and I was inside. All of a sudden we heard an ambulance going by. The local hospital was two blocks away. Every time we'd hear an ambulance siren, we'd hop on our bikes and follow it to the hospital, hoping to see some blood and gore.

"When I heard the ambulance, I also heard Jimmy yell through the front door, 'Hey, Bobby! There's an ambulance. Let's go!'

"There I was, sitting with Carol Lind and debating about going despite what my mother had told me. The ambulance won out. I told my baby sister to just stay in the house and I'd be back in a few minutes. Then I ran out, jumped on my bike, and followed Jimmy and his friends to the hospital.

"When I got back, Mama was already home. Carol Lind was crying and pointing at me. Mama got a belt and it's the last whipping I can ever remember getting from her. She didn't apologize like she used to do when she was drinking. She gave me a talking-to instead."

At Lee Street, there was always a kitchen filled with recovering alcoholics when Bobby came home from school each day. Dot would be right in the middle of them talking about the Twelve Steps and how to live sober. Bobby always got a cheerful greeting and someone would offer him something to eat or drink. Then he'd usually have to step over someone dozing in the hallway or on the stairs as he headed to his bedroom to do his homework.

"I knew it was an unusual way to live," he commented. "But that's just the way it was."

Bobby recalled that while he was still living in the house, an incident occurred that brought back memories of his father's drinking and the strange way he would act at times.

"I was asleep in my bedroom late one night when this guy knocked on my door. I remembered my dad had brought him home a few nights before very drunk. This guy said to me, 'Bobby, you've got to do me a favor. You've got to come outside with me. I think there's some trouble going on.'

"For some reason, I grabbed the hunting rifle my dad had bought for me, loaded it, and followed the guy downstairs. Nobody else in the house was awake. We went outside and he started looking around. I was getting a little nervous. He turned to me and said, 'I saw two strange guys hanging around over there. I think we just scared them away. Good job, Bobby.' I said to him, 'Golly. I'm sure glad we did.'

"We went back inside and I went back to bed. A few minutes later, the guy knocked on my door again. He said, 'Bobby, hurry up and get your gun. I think they're back!'

"We went outside and he pointed to a car. He said, 'They're in that car!' We went sneaking over and I pointed my rifle while he yanked open the car door. The lights went on in the car but there was nobody in there. Just then, another more sober guy came out of the house, walked over to us, and I told him what's going on. He started to laugh and said, 'Your friend here has the DTs. He's been hallucinating.'

"He walked the guy into the house and woke up my dad to take care of him. I just snuck back upstairs and tried to go to sleep. But I finally understood what the DTs meant."

The next day Bobby moved into the log cabin his father had built in the backyard.

While the Mooneys' sons each had a variety of memories concerning their parents' early sobriety and their dedication to helping other alcoholics get well, it was their daughter, Carol Lind, who grew up totally surrounded by that environment. She had been born into her mom and dad's whole new world of recovery and the whirlwind of activity that went with it.

"The one thing I always knew," the pretty, blond-haired lady fondly recalled, "was that I was loved very deeply by both my parents. In fact, my mother rarely went anywhere without me. She dragged me all over with her—to counseling sessions she had with her sponsees, to all kinds of meetings, even to the beauty parlor during those rare moments when she would take time out for herself.

"And my dad—I knew I was the apple of his eye. I remember how he loved sitting me on his knee and telling me stories. I would run to him and kiss and hug him whenever he came into the room. And when they both got very busy trying to help other alcoholics get well, I always had plenty of babysitters at the house. So I never, ever felt unloved."

Carol Lind was once asked what it was like growing up in a house filled with alcoholics in various stages of recovery. Like her brothers, who had experienced the fallout from their parents' disease, she said it seemed rather normal.

"It probably wouldn't seem normal to most people," she explained, "but all that was just part of my life. I've seen my mother run after drunken people who were out of control. I've seen her grab others to help her hold someone down when they were convulsing. I know the smell of vomit and urine from addicts who couldn't control themselves. Also back then, we didn't have the medications and stuff we have now so there was a lot more physical ramifications."

One of her earliest memories of the many events she experienced at Lee Street happened one Christmas morning when the patients almost ruined a special surprise Santa had for her. It was an incident she often teased her mother about later on.

"I was always kind of a tomboy," she said, laughing. "Much to my parents' dismay I loved horses and cowboys more than dolls and tea sets. I was around five or six years old that Christmas, and

I wanted a Johnny West set. It was a cowboy set with horses, a red barn, and some animals. I had seen it in a store window.

"That Christmas Eve I was so excited I couldn't sleep. It was probably around 1 a.m. when I got up and went down to the kitchen. There was a housekeeper there cleaning up. I said to her, 'Has Santa come yet?' She replied, 'No, Santa Claus hasn't come. He's not going to come until you go to sleep for the night.'

"When the housekeeper turned around, I walked quietly toward our large playroom, where my father had put up our Christmas tree and decorated it with everyone's help. The room had swinging doors, like saloon doors almost. I pushed one open slightly and peeked in. There were twenty patients or so sitting on the floor playing with my Johnny West set. I remember getting so mad at them."

Later in life, when Carol Lind thought about that incident, she realized that most of the patients in the playroom at Lee Street that Christmas morning were the same age emotionally as she was at the time.

John and Dot's daughter said she could still smell the aromas of the Southern cooking that filled the kitchen in the afternoons as her mother prepared the delicious buffet dinner she served to the patients every single night.

"My mother loved to cook and she was a great cook," Carol Lind bragged. "I can still see her frying chicken and pork chops and talking and counseling patients at the same time. We had a kidney-shaped, self-standing counter in the middle of the large kitchen, and people would be sitting around it on bar stools.

"I remember there was always a roomful of people asking my mother question after question. She would either know the answers or she would shout, 'Look it up in the Big Book!'

"My daddy had the chair at the head of the big dining room table where the telephone was because he was always on the phone. People were either calling to ask him questions like they did with my mother, or he'd be checking on some really sick patient who was still in the hospital. He'd also get calls inviting him to speak at meetings or big AA conventions. I'll never forget how busy it was there all of the time."

Aside from the busyness and the drama that was an integral part of Lee Street, there was something else that stood out—something else that both the Mooneys' young daughter and everyone who spent any amount of time there could see and feel. John and Dot called it "unconditional love"—the very special caring one alcoholic has for another.

"Yes, I really did feel like there was something very special about my house," Carol Lind explained. "When you came into my house, you couldn't go from one room to the other without getting a hug, without somebody telling you they loved you, without somebody asking if you're okay.

"My friends loved coming to my house. That's where everybody wanted to be because it was so different in a nice and friendly kind of way. The patients were so happy to see my friends, and my friends felt so good and special about that. Yes, there was definitely something real special about it."

Still, the pretty lady from Statesboro had to admit there were times she would try the patience of some patients at Lee Street without realizing it. There was one particular lady at the house by the name of Martha Jones who loved the seven-year-old Carol Lind but still found her to be "a pain in the ass" at times.

"I remember Martha real well," the Mooneys' daughter said, grinning. "She took her meetings very seriously. She'd make sure all the patients at the house were in the living room at three o'clock sharp every afternoon to start their AA meeting on time.

"I'd arrive home from school and come busting in without giving any thought as to what was going on. I'd throw my books on the floor and head for my aquarium next to the wall to feed my fish. Then I'd sit down and talk to the fish. It must have been very annoying to some of the people who were trying to hear what was being said at the meeting.

"But my mom and dad never told me, 'You can't come in here

when there's a meeting going on.' They said it was my house and I could go anywhere I wanted anytime I wanted to. I guess I never thought about how it might bother people."

It only made matters worse when Carol Lind got her first pony.

"I named him Bobo, after John Wayne's horse, and we kept him in the backyard," she explained. "When the weather was really nice, my mother would keep the outside doors to the living room wide open. They faced the yard. Sometimes I had a difficult time controlling Bobo and we'd ride right into the living room, again while a meeting was going on.

"One of the funniest things I remember was the day a squirrel followed me in. It stopped right in the middle of the room and seemed to look around at everybody. Suddenly the room got very quiet. Then I heard someone say, 'Hey, look. It's a squirrel!' Then I heard someone else say, 'Thank God. I thought I was hallucinating.' Everyone roared with laughter, including my mother."

Carol Lind said there was one other funny story she remembered that her mother talked about for years. It was the result of what the young girl constantly heard at Lee Street and also at all the AA meetings she went to with her parents.

"For some reason I had a lot of fear about going into the second grade at school," she explained. "In the first grade, the teacher carried your lunch tray to your table. In the second grade, you had to do it yourself, and I was afraid I'd drop it and make a fool out of myself.

"My father thought it would give me a lot of self-confidence and make me feel more comfortable if I learned everybody's name in my class. So he sent me off to school one day with a tape recorder that I could pass around and have everybody speak their name into it. Well, all my classmates said their names and when it got back to me, I said, 'Hi, I'm Carol Lind Mooney and I'm an alcoholic.'

"Believe it or not, my teacher called my mom and dad, saying, 'This is devastating. Your daughter is in second grade calling herself an alcoholic.' Of course, my parents thought it was hilarious. They laughed and talked about it the rest of their lives."

Despite all she had seen and experienced at Lee Street and elsewhere growing up, Carol Lind Mooney, like her brothers Jimmy and Bobby, became an alcoholic and drug addict herself. Fortunately, after going through fourteen rehabs and making other attempts to stop her addiction, she took her last drink at the age of twenty-one and has been clean and sober since June 28, 1982. She went on to follow in her parents' footsteps. Today she counsels women alcoholics and drug addicts in the same home where she grew up and where it all began—Lee Street—which is now a recovery house.

Some say alcoholism is a family disease, that it has its origins in the genes. While science has yet to prove this proposition, there are untold indications pointing in that direction—including the Mooney family itself.

While John hadn't noticed the disease rearing its ugly head in his offspring as yet, he was doing everything he could to fight the malady wherever he went. He was not only continuing his medical practice and tending to patients at Lee Street at the same time, he was now speaking all over the country, even returning to the drug prison in Lexington to express his gratitude for finding his sobriety there.

A letter he received on January 21, 1966, from Dr. Robert W. Rasor, the Lexington facility's medical director, says it all:

Dear Dr. Mooney,

We all enjoyed your latest visit to the hospital in December and your help to the many patients who had the opportunity of meeting with you. I wanted to let you know that we are deeply grateful for the time that you take to return to the hospital, and to speak with many of the patients who are so in need of encouragement and inspiration.

It is always a source of great pleasure to me to learn from individuals who have themselves been here in the hospital and who have been able to find a way of life without resorting to their drugs.

I hope you will continue to return as often as you can, and we sincerely appreciate your support of the program of the hospital.

Sincerely yours.

Like her husband, Dot Mooney also enjoyed doing Twelve-Step work because she knew it was saving her life. And also like John, she never thought twice about not charging for anything at Lee Street.

"I was getting so much out of helping our fellow alcoholics," she would say, "that I never paid any attention to what it was costing us. For example, I just loved being in the kitchen with a bunch of crying women. One would start crying over some sad story and another would join her. Before you knew it, I'd be crying right along with them.

"I'd get out a few bushels of butter beans and we'd sit there all day preparing them and talking and crying while we were getting things ready for supper. It was good for me and it was good for them. I wouldn't take anything for those days."

Dot said one day their accountant, Earl Dabbs, called with some news she found very disturbing. He said if they didn't make any changes in the way they were operating at Lee Street, they were headed for bankruptcy. He said they couldn't keep feeding everybody and paying for their medical expenses without going broke. He concluded by saying that if they were going to keep treating alcoholics at their home, they had to start charging them something.

"When he said that, it scared me nearly half to death," she recalled. "I always faced the horror of going bankrupt when John and I were drinking and taking so many drugs. I had nightmares over it. I don't know how we managed to keep our heads above water. But now when I felt we were doing better, just the thought of charging someone to stay at my home really bothered me. It was one of the hardest things I had to face."

Earl Dabbs finally sat down with John, who was both his friend and a client. He laid out the physician's financial problems in full detail. The accountant explained that John was not only paying to house, feed, counsel, and care for more than thirty alcoholics living at his home, he also now had to hire some full-time staff people to clean, help cook, and handle security on a twenty-four-hour basis.

Earl pointed out that his client was also spending a considerable amount of money traveling to AA conventions and for other related activities, as well as still paying for rooms at the Norris Hotel for some of his alcoholic patients. Not only was all this very costly, but it was taking time away from his medical practice, which could be even more successful and profitable were he there more often. The accountant's advice was to begin charging his Lee Street patients a little something to start with and then gradually raise the fee, particularly for new patients who came for treatment.

"I was running so fast at the time," the physician would explain, "that I wasn't paying attention to the simple facts my accountant was explaining to me. However, when you're sober and people bring things to your attention, you can see them quite clearly. So I realized I had to follow my accountant's advice or else."

Patients at Lee Street started to be charged five dollars a day, which included their medical care, food, and board. It didn't come close to covering the costs. Gradually the charge became more realistic, rising to six hundred dollars for a four-week stay. As more staff workers had to be hired, the charge went to eight hundred dollars a month. What kept the costs down to some degree was the fact that John was the entire medical staff with assistance from Dallas Cason at times and also from Dot, who had been a nurse.

Dallas remembered how she would bounce back and forth between Dr. Mooney's medical office and the Lee Street house to help treat his alcoholic patients.

"If they needed a chest X-ray," she said, "I'd pick them up at the house, bring them to the office, and then bring them back. If they needed an injection, I'd give it to them along with special things like IVs. And I'd help Dot with any special medications that we used mainly for detoxification.

"One day I went hunting for this particular patient in that crowded house, and someone told me he was upstairs in the closet. I said, 'Closet!?' They laughed and led me upstairs to a walk-in closet. I said to the patient, 'I'm sure sorry they had to put you in here.' The man replied, 'Oh, I'm glad I'm in here. This is the only private place in the whole house.'

"Maybe it wasn't that funny, but I had to laugh."

Discussing the evolution and growth of their Lee Street adventure, John once explained, "I had just delivered a baby in an emergency procedure at the hospital so it was around three a.m. by the time I got home. There was this lady sitting on the back steps shelling peas. She said she was also part of the security detail, watching over the kitchen. She happened to be our first all-night employee. That's when I realized the patient load had increased so much that the facility which had been our home had now taken us over. As a result, I now knew we needed a more organized structure to make it a more effective place for recovery."

Reconfiguring the house wasn't all that hard to do as far as the layout of the building was concerned. Since the large, oval-shaped bar in the middle of the kitchen was the center of activity, it was also a natural divider for keeping the men on one side of the house and the women on the other side. That helped solve the problem of separating the sexes.

As for the recovery program that was being developed, sometimes on a hit-or-miss basis, it would begin in the dining room. That's where patients would detox under Dot's beautiful chandelier.

As they began to get well physically, they would become involved in comfortable "family style" sessions in which John and Dot and some new staff members shared their own experiences, encouraged patients to share their situations, and counseled those still filled with fear, guilt, and remorse, mainly using the suggestions found in AA's Big Book. John became increasingly convinced that this "family style" setup was one of the most valuable things Lee Street had to offer—in addition to taking patients to outside AA meetings.

And when it came to keeping tabs on everyone in the house, John left most of that to his wife: "Since Dot did most of the cooking and much of the counseling, she also did most of the supervising during the day. We used our new staff people to help her and then supervise the place at night. Most of our patients were really dedicated to staying sober, so we had very few problems in the house even though we treated almost six hundred alcoholics and addicts over a five-year period."

Another reason there was so little trouble at Lee Street were the rules John and Dot strictly enforced as more patients came there for treatment. Upon admittance, for example, everyone was carefully checked for any hidden booze or pills or other substances. Also, personal property and other valuables were either given to a family member or carefully noted and stored away.

Despite the rules, there were still occasional misunderstandings. Dot often shared one of the more humorous incidents: "This rather obese fellow arrived quite inebriated. We admitted him, helped him get undressed, and went through his few belongings. He had nothing of any value except a few dollars in his wallet, which we let him keep. The next morning he started claiming he had six hundred dollars with him and now it was missing. We showed him the list of what he had when he arrived, but he wouldn't listen. He said somebody must have taken his money.

"The fellow got so upset he decided to leave. He sat down to get dressed. He put on one shoe but couldn't get his foot into the other one. There was something stuck inside. He reached in and pulled out his six hundred dollars. He forgot he had hidden it in his shoe to keep it safe. I think that convinced him he needed help because he decided to stay."

John used to tell a similar story about a very rich gentleman who had a serious problem with both alcohol and drugs: "We got a call one night from this wealthy guy who wanted us to send an airplane to pick him up at some private airport seven hundred miles away. After checking his credentials and references, we sent the plane with a nurse and attendant on board. He finally arrived, very drunk, so we put him in the dining room to detox.

"The next morning he came to in a panic. He told Dot that when he drove to the airport the night before, he had five thousand dollars in his pocket. He demanded to know what happened to the money. Now, we had searched this guy's fancy clothes, including his hat and his wallet, to make sure he had no booze or drugs with him. We certainly didn't find the five thousand dollars he was ranting about. But he kept insisting he had brought it with him.

"Finally, we had someone call this fellow's wife. She confirmed her husband had taken the money with him when he drove to the private airport. We suggested she go to the airport, find his car, and check it. Sure enough the money had fallen out of his pocket and was lying all over the floor of the car. That's when we put in another rule: that patients could not bring large sums of money with them, and, if a family member brought them for treatment, the patient had to turn over to them all their valuables. Most alcoholics have very bad memories, especially when it comes to money."

One of the things Dot discovered was that women were much cleverer than men when it came to hiding alcohol or drugs, particularly pills. She would say laughingly, "I'd find their drugs under the powder puff in their makeup compact, in the toes of their stockings, in the lining of their coats, or even sewn into the hems in their underwear. One woman who came in had pills in the tube of her douche bag and another had them stuffed into all her tampons.

"I would also check the lining in their baggage and find prescriptions for drugs from their medical doctor, their psychiatrist, even their gynecologist. And they wanted us to fill them all. I'd say, 'Sure, honey, after we've detoxed you from all the other stuff you already have in you.' Later I'd apologize for telling them a fib that was for their own good. We rarely filled any of their prescriptions. We found they didn't need them."

Another important thing that John and his wife learned through their experiences at Lee Street was that the public stigma associated with alcoholism and drug addiction, which still exists today, caused many people to deny their illness and become sicker and sicker as a result.

"We discovered that most addicts really need treatment two or three years before they actually seek it," the physician would explain. "Most alcoholics and drug addicts will fight it to the bitter end, just like I did. They'll deny it to the death. That's why by the time they arrived at Lee Street, usually being sent by a doctor or a psychiatrist or a family member, they were often very, very ill."

As alcoholism and drug addiction continued to grow like a plague across this country, as it is still doing today, inquiries from afflicted addicts poured into Lee Street. Also, more and more doctors who had heard about the successful treatment facility in Statesboro wanted to send their alcoholic patients there. This attention only exacerbated the space problems at the house.

In the fall of 1968, John and Dot decided to add a five-bedroom wing to the house. They hired an architect and filed their plans with the city. While Honey and Bill Bowen, along with a few others, cheered them on, most of their neighbors were not quite so pleased. In fact, they were downright upset. When they learned about the planned expansion, they petitioned the city of Statesboro to deny the building permit, stating that they did not like the idea of putting "some kind of big alcoholic place" in the middle of a nice residential neighborhood.

Understanding their neighbors' feelings, John and Dot promptly admitted their error, canceled the plans, and notified their neighbors of the decision. The couple continued to operate as usual, trying to make the best out of a very tight and often difficult situation.

Earl Dabbs had been keeping a close watch on all these developments. Like Statesboro's mayor, Bill Bowen, and his wife, Honey, the accountant was almost awed by what he would refer to as "the resurrection of Dr. John Mooney." And now observing all that the physician and his wife were doing to save the lives of other people suffering from the same addiction moved him deeply.

Earl knew that something had to be done to solve the problem at Lee Street, so he set about doing it.

CHAPTER FOURTEEN

The Miracle of Recovery

FOR MOST PEOPLE IN AMERICA AND EVEN AROUND THE WORLD, drinking alcoholic beverages is a pleasurable social activity usually undertaken on special occasions such as holidays, weddings, anniversaries, and similar events. Various forms of alcohol have also been a staple for more than twelve thousand years in medicine, religious ceremonies, and even funeral offerings.

Although there have been stories of madness, chaos, and degradation related to alcohol and drugs down through the years, the first serious chronicles of uncontrollable drinking related to poor health and premature death didn't seem to appear until the 1700s. And it wasn't until 1849 that the term "alcoholism" was first coined by a Swedish physician named Magnus Huss.

Several decades earlier, however, in 1810, Benjamin Rush, a Philadelphia physician and a signer of the Declaration of Independence, was said to be the first formulator of a disease concept as it pertained to heavy drinking. He was also the first to propose that "sober houses" be created for the special treatment of drunkards. It was around the same time that a man named Samuel

Woodward, who was a temperance orator and the superintendent of a Massachusetts insane asylum, began touting his own theory that habitual drunkenness was caused by a malfunction of the body.

The line of thinking staked out by Rush and Woodward was that drunks and tosspots could not be treated successfully on a voluntary basis—that they required legal restraint in a "well conducted environment." This launched the inebriate asylum movement in the 1800s and led to states like New York, Pennsylvania, Massachusetts, Minnesota, and California opening subsidized facilities, primarily for destitute alcoholics, or street derelicts as they were called back then.

The inebriate asylum movement also spawned dozens of private sanitariums in the early 1900s such as Towns Hospital in New York City that over the years catered to and treated well-to-do and "celebrity drunkards," such as actor John Barrymore and Irish poet Brendan Behan. But the movement for both public and private treatment for alcoholism failed at that time for two main reasons.

First, physicians working in the so-called addiction treatment field in those years could not produce a strictly medical "cure" for alcoholism or drug abuse. Second, they totally dispensed with the concepts of spirituality and the therapeutic necessity of fellowship among those suffering from the same malady. They relied totally on recuperation by bed rest, a healthy diet, and therapeutic baths or hydrotherapy.

The protocol of hydrotherapy has been used in occupational therapy for many years. It encompasses a broad range of approaches and therapeutic methods involving the physical properties of water such as temperature and pressure that can stimulate blood circulation and treat the symptoms of certain diseases. It was often used in the late 1800s and early 1900s for the detoxification of alcoholics. It was believed to help relieve the states of delirium and depression and "awaken" brain function.

With poor results being reported from the inebriate asylum

movement, few state legislatures could be persuaded that the building of costly treatment facilities was worth the price. Many private facilities also closed their doors, except for a few that were still used as "fancy drying-out places."

It wasn't until Alcoholics Anonymous came along in 1935 and offered a program that focused on all three aspects of the disease of alcoholism—the physical, the mental, and the spiritual—that true and lasting recovery from addiction was made possible.

John and Dot Mooney came to recognize this possibility in their own lives and turned it into a reality. They also came to see that the vast majority of alcoholics could find sobriety by simply dedicating themselves 100 percent to working AA's Twelve Steps to Recovery in their lives.

In an attempt to help others find sobriety, Dr. John Mooney Jr. in particular came to realize there was a small percentage of very sick alcoholics and drug addicts who required special medical and often psychological help for their advanced physical and mental problems. The process he and his wife developed at Lee Street was designed specifically to get addicts physically and mentally well enough so that they could move out of the house and live on their own with the support and fellowship of the spiritual program of Alcoholics Anonymous.

But now there was no more room at the inn, so to speak. It was the summer of 1968, and Lee Street was bursting at the seams. As the physician once said, "You couldn't squeeze another person in there with a shoehorn." And it bothered him and his wife greatly since inquiries and requests for treatment were arriving almost daily.

Shortly after they scrapped their plans to expand their home one more time because of their neighbors' complaints, John dropped by to see his accountant to discuss his current financial situation.

Earl Dabbs remembered asking his friend that day, "John, does it ever bother you to have so many people in your house?"

He said Dr. Mooney told him, "No, Earl. I'm just so damn glad

I'm not one of them anymore. I used to be. Maybe that's why it doesn't bother me a bit. I step around them, I step over them, and I do whatever I can to help them. In fact, I wish we could help more."

Then Earl replied, "What you need to do, John, is to build a hospital to take care of them."

His client was stunned at first by the suggestion but then asked, "How the hell do I do that?"

The accountant explained that he had worked very closely with the Small Business Administration on a number of projects and developed a close friendship with a man in Atlanta named Ed Tingle, who was a loan officer for the SBA. He said his friend was in charge of a special undertaking called the Local Development Program, which was designed for new start-up businesses.

"I've put together a number of nursing home transactions with Ed Tingle," Earl went on to say, "and I never gave him a bad loan. The projects I brought him were only the ones that I believed in, and they all turned out very well. I think there might be an SBA program out there that could help us get this job done, John. So why don't you and I do a little exploring. What do you say?"

The physician was absolutely lost for words. He knew he himself couldn't borrow a nickel, not with the bad credit record he had rung up. And surely the fact that he had been in prison on a drug felony charge wasn't going to help. All of this could be nothing but a bunch of hot air.

Then as he started to think more about it, he became aware once again of the most important thing that had happened in his life as a result of his time at the narcotics hospital in Lexington and his work at Lee Street. He had become reunited with someone who had always been on his side—something that all the money in the world couldn't buy. He had found a Higher Power in his life, a God of his understanding.

John suddenly sensed deep within himself that if God wanted to build a hospital for all his drunks, then maybe He was planning to use Earl Dabbs to get the job done. That's when he reached out, shook his accountant's hand, and said, "If you can do this, my friend, you'll be helping an awful lot of people who need help."

Over the next few weeks, the two men met to discuss such things as the number of patients John thought he could have on a steady basis, what the charges might be, the cost of staff and medical equipment and other expenditures related to running a hospital. They even had an architect friend of theirs, Edwin Eckles, develop a rough design and a ballpark estimate for land and construction costs.

Dot became so enthralled with the idea of having a hospital where they would have room to treat their patients with more comfort and dignity that she began running all over town looking for just the right place to build such a facility. She soon found what she called the ideal spot—an eleven-acre, tree-covered site on Jones Mill Road, only a short drive from Lee Street. John and Earl both agreed with her choice. They made the owner an offer on the land, and he accepted it after Dot told him what they planned to build on it.

"When I ran the numbers," Earl recalled, "the project came to over one million dollars. But the numbers also showed that such a treatment facility could produce a profit. I mentioned what we were doing to our mayor, Bill Bowen, and a few more of our friends, and all they did was smile. As much as they respected Dr. Mooney and admired his recovery, I think they thought I was wasting my time. As the mayor put it, 'John's come a long way, but he can't borrow that kind of money.'"

Still, that assessment didn't deter the determined accountant. He called Ed Tingle and took him out for a steak dinner. His goal was to get an oral commitment if possible before filling out all the forms and plodding through all the SBA red tape.

"I've got a very special project that I believe can work out quite well," was how Earl started the conversation that evening. "There are some hurdles we may have to jump over, but in the end I think it will be worthwhile."

Then, after briefly outlining the proposed hospital plan and its tentative costs, the accountant told the loan officer all about Dr. John Mooney—that the written application involving his personal history would reveal he once had a serious alcohol and drug abuse problem, had been indicted on drug felony charges, went to prison, but had been clean and sober now for more than eight years.

He also told Tingle all about the fine work the physician and his wife were doing to save the lives of addicts who came to them from Statesboro, as well as from many different cities and states. Then he took a deep breath and waited for the SBA official to reply.

"Well, all that's all right with me," Ed Tingle said rather warmly. "What we look at is what he's all about today and that sounds very impressive."

Earl waited another moment, hoping to hear what he really wanted to hear. Then he heard it.

"If the numbers work out like you say," Ed concluded, "then it looks like we got a deal. Go ahead and put it together."

That's when the real work began. According to the rules and regulations of the Small Business Administration, any company seeking a loan under the Local Development Program had to raise 10 percent of the total cost of the project locally. That meant John Mooney had to raise $100,000 before any other monies would be available. The rest of the financial plan called for the SBA to lend $450,000 and a Statesboro bank to lend the other $450,000.

"The local bank loan wasn't the problem," Earl clearly recalled. "The president of Statesboro's First Federal Savings and Loan was a friend of ours. Also, the bank's loan would be secured by the land and structures on it. For the hundred thousand dollars, we had to find some 'angels' who believed their investment would eventually be paid back through any profits from the proposed hospital."

First, however, two separate corporations had to be formed—a development company they called "Statesboro Development Company," and another entity that would be the actual hospital built by the development company. That entity needed a name.

Now that Dot had found the location for the hospital, she was eager to find the right name for it. She once explained exactly how the name "Willingway" came about.

"We couldn't think of anything ourselves at first, so we offered a five-dollar prize to anyone at the house who could come up with a suitable name. There were a lot of proposals bandied about, but nothing we thought appropriate.

"One night John and I were sitting in the kitchen talking about it. He said any old name would do since whatever it was would become significant as more and more people heard it and repeated it, like one of our favorite places in West Virginia called the Greenbriar. He then suggested that since the property we had picked to build on was covered with pinewoods, why didn't we call it something like 'Willingwoods'?

"I really liked that idea because it made me think of people being willing to come here for treatment. And then I thought, when they got here, they were also willing for us to show them the way to get sober. If you're willing, there's a way. That's how John and I agreed to call the hospital 'Willingway.' Neither of us got the five dollars."

Now that there was an agreement on the property and loan deals with the SBA and the bank, John and Earl got busy trying to raise the $100,000 needed for closure.

"The first place you start," said the experienced accountant, "is with the people you're doing business with. Our architect, Edwin Eckles, was the first to invest, followed by John's attorney. Then came some people at the drug companies John was doing business with again, only now legitimately.

"There were a few rather wealthy people he had treated over at Lee Street who, when they heard about the project, wanted to be part of it. There's a bit of a humorous story connected to that, I mean, people he treated who wanted to invest.

"We went to see this pretty successful doctor in South Carolina whom John once had as a patient at his house. The guy was still sober and doing real well. We got there kind of late. He took us into his garage and opened the trunk of his car. It was filled with cash, I mean thousands of dollars. I don't remember how much he gave us to invest, but it was a whole lot.

"I had a hunch it was money this doctor had never paid taxes on. But that was none of our business. We weren't concerned about his taxes. We were concerned about coming up with $100,000. So we took the money as an investment and went ahead and put the rest of the project together."

It was near the end of 1969 before all the paperwork was completed, the funds made available to the new Statesboro Development Company, and all the architectural and construction plans approved. Actual work on the Willingway project didn't get under way, however, until April 1970. When the hospital finally opened on August 12, 1971, it was the only facility in the state licensed by the Georgia State Board of Health for the exclusive purpose of detoxification and long-term treatment of alcoholics and drug addicts.

While waiting for all the pieces to fall into place, John kept himself busy, not only at his medical practice and at Lee Street, but also by getting involved in other activities he felt were both important and meaningful. For example, the 1960s had brought forced racial integration to the South and, with it, a great deal of tension and resentment. The physician was constantly looking for ways to help African Americans find recovery from addiction just as he had helped so many others. That's when he found an old friend and army veteran like himself to join him in that cause.

He was Lonnie Simmons, also a Statesboro native and a decorated war hero who had become addicted to alcohol and drugs while fighting in the Korean War and in Vietnam. A warm and kind black man, Lonnie and John hadn't known each other growing up but had much in common, including serving as paratroopers in the Eighty-Second Airborne Division and the fact that the physician's father had delivered Lonnie.

After leaving the army's Special Forces unit, Lonnie returned to Statesboro and continued to drink up all the money he had saved while in the service. When things got really bad, he'd check into the Veterans Administration hospital in Augusta to get detoxed.

One day, a psychiatrist at the VA hospital said to him, "Lonnie, there's a drunk doctor in your own home town of Statesboro who's now sober and helping people just like you. Why don't you go see him?"

The decorated veteran had several reasons to follow the psychiatrist's advice. "First of all," he said, "I was broke and had to find a way to get back on my feet. Second, my family was trying to put me into a mental institution because I had gotten so bad. And then when I heard the name Dr. Mooney, I recognized it from around town and also remembered my mother told me his father had delivered me as a baby. So, after another bad bout with alcohol and drugs, I decided to go see him.

"Dr. John put me right into Bulloch County Hospital to detox. Before he discharged me a week later, he insisted I come to his office every day so we could talk about my addiction and meet others who had the same problem. I was allowed back in my home as long as I went to see Dr. John. He and I soon became very good friends, maybe because we had so much in common even though I was black and he was white. I could tell right from the start that the color of your skin didn't make a damn bit of difference to him.

"We met in a small room in the front of his office with a handful of other alcoholics and drug addicts. At that time, no black people were allowed in any of the recovery meetings around town, only there at Dr. John's office. It was a difficult period in the

South back then as far as integration was concerned. It took a few years, but eventually all the recovery meetings in Statesboro and throughout the South became totally integrated.

"For almost two years, I was the only black person there trying to stay sober. Once in a while, Dr. John would ask me to invite some of the black orderlies at the hospital he knew drank too much and took drugs. He also sent me after the local black jail keeper. He wanted my help to reach out to the black community. He would say that sobriety wasn't just for white people, it was for everybody—that the disease of alcoholism and drug addiction kills you regardless of your skin color."

After Lonnie was sober a few years, he received a call from an old army buddy who worked for the Georgia Department of Corrections in Reidsville, the hard-core prison where John Mooney almost landed. Lonnie's buddy was in charge of the prison guards and said the state had been mandated by the federal government to integrate the entire correctional system. He offered his friend a job there.

So in 1968 the decorated war hero became the first African American to walk into Reidsville State Penitentiary as a prison guard instead of as an inmate. He would always tell everybody that it was because Dr. John helped him get sober.

Meanwhile, the Statesboro surgeon kept seeking ways to carry the message of sobriety more effectively into the minority communities and the impoverished areas of his hometown. In 1970, he and several others active in recovery met with U.S. Senator Harold Hughes (D-IA), who some years earlier had publicly admitted he was a recovered alcoholic. The discussions they had, together with a series of committee hearings the senator held on the growing national crisis of addiction, led to the establishment of the National Institute on Alcohol Abuse and Alcoholism. One of the aims of the NIAAA was to provide funds to state governments to establish and support addiction recovery programs.

With the help of some political friends in Atlanta who had come to know and respect the sober physician, John managed to get an NIAAA grant from the state to establish a small recovery center in Statesboro called the Bulloch Residence Center. It was designed for both inpatient and outpatient care and was aimed primarily at helping poor and underprivileged addicts in the community find recovery.

It was serendipitous that Lonnie Simmons came to dislike his job as a prison guard around this same time. He decided to leave Reidsville and return to Statesboro. Upon hearing this, Dr. Mooney asked him to serve as a counselor at the new center, becoming part of a five-person team that included a nurse, a social worker, a minister, and himself as the physician. Lonnie immediately agreed, and with his assistance, the center went on to help many sick addicts, both black and white, who couldn't afford treatment elsewhere.

The nurse who was part of that team, Nancy Waters, well remembers those times and the hard work Lonnie Simmons and her good friend Dr. Mooney invested to make it a success.

"I had known Dr. Mooney practically all of my life, even though he was some years older," the soft-spoken nurse explained. "He had delivered my children and, knowing I was a nurse, called me after he had gotten his medical license back in 1960 to help out at his office.

"Dallas Cason and I were already well acquainted, so it was a very comfortable situation assisting her or filling in for her at times. That's when the doctor and I and his wife, Dot, became very close friends.

"I remember the first week I worked for him and saw how many alcoholics he was treating. He was not only putting them in beds in two of the exam rooms in the back of his office, but he was also detoxing them wherever they were—at a motel, in the Norris Hotel, even in jail. And it didn't make any difference whether they were black or white, which is what I really admired about him since there was a lot of fuss concerning integration back then.

"There were times when someone would be so inebriated and couldn't get to his office that he would go see them himself or send Dallas or me. I'll never forget the day he sent me over to this really low-class motel to give detox medication to a man who had been so drunk for more than a week that he couldn't get out of bed.

"Here I was riding through town in my car with two syringes lying on the seat next to me loaded with phenobarbital. I began thinking, 'What if the police stop me and I've got these two loaded syringes? What am I going to do? How am I going to get out of it?'

"I've given detox medications to black folks in jail and white folks at the Norris Hotel. It didn't matter. Dr. Mooney had wealthy alcoholics coming to his house to be treated as well as the bottom of the barrel all over town. It made me feel good helping him to try saving the lives of all these people suffering from this terrible addiction."

Nurse Waters said she knew a lot about the disease of alcoholism since it ran in her own family. That's also why she enjoyed her work at John's medical office and later at the Bulloch Residence Center. She also helped treat alcoholics at Lee Street where, as she said, she became part of the Mooney family.

As if all these developments weren't enough to keep the energetic surgeon's plate overflowing, there was yet another venture that had always attracted his interest—flying. It was one he had never pursued, however, due to his drinking and drugging. But now he was sober.

In the summer of 1968, John watched his son Jimmy receive his pilot's license and solo for the first time. That turned his itch into a scratch, and despite his wife's words of caution, he started taking flying lessons.

One of the character traits the talented doctor had that never really changed was the excitement and enthusiasm he could generate when facing a new challenge. When he got interested in something—whether it be carpentry, photography, or fancy cars—he jumped in full bore. And that's how it was with flying.

John not only earned his pilot's license in a matter of months but also, despite his tight finances, managed to buy a brand-new Piper Cherokee 180 in 1968. Before long he was flying off to AA meetings and conventions in towns and cities far beyond States-boro. At first Dot was reluctant to join him. But he became such a good pilot in the eyes of all who flew with him that she soon developed the confidence to hop aboard and go along for the exciting ride.

While Dot tried to spend time with her husband whenever she could, it was not always possible. She had her own load of responsibilities to handle both at Lee Street and with her family. The boys were pretty much on their own by now, but Carol Lind was still a child and needed her mother's attention.

At the same time, Dot was in need of her husband's attention, and with his almost impossible schedule, she was getting less and less of it. She could feel her resentment smoldering. She knew and preached to others that resentments can lead an alcoholic back to a drink. So she tried to handle it as best she could, mainly by working closely with the patients at the house.

One young lady in particular, Corliss Gibbons, helped Dot a great deal. Corliss was one of the last patients Dot and John took into Lee Street before the hospital was built. She had been drinking and abusing drugs since she was a teenager and had reached a very low bottom in her life. Dot sensed she was ready to surrender and did everything she could from the moment she entered treatment to help the young woman recover. Perhaps she also did it because she knew it would lessen the resentment she herself was still trying to overcome.

As it turned out, not only did Corliss find sobriety at Lee Street, she and Dot became very close friends and remained so for the rest of their lives.

"Dot Mooney saved my life," the young woman would always say when describing their relationship.

"My parents had disowned me because I was such a bad alcoholic and drug addict. But then they heard about this place in Statesboro that treated the worst alcoholics imaginable and shipped me off there. I was about four or five months pregnant at the time from my second husband, who was also a terrible drunk.

"I remember waking up on a cot in the upstairs hallway. I was a pitiable sight. I felt so alone and unwanted. I probably deserved feeling like that because of all the terrible things I had done and all the people I had hurt through my drinking and drugging. But to tell the truth, I had never felt loved or accepted anywhere in my whole life. All that changed with Dot and the other people at Lee Street.

"I was there a few days when Dot said she wanted to take me to a meeting. I remember telling her, 'Dot, I'm just too filthy to go. I really need a shower if you're going to take me anywhere.' She looked at me and smiled and said, 'Yeah, honey, you're right. You do need a shower. You really are filthy.'

"I was so weak she had to help me get up. As we walked down the hallway to the bathroom, she could see that I was very shaky. She turned on the shower, helped me off with my nightgown, and put me in. When she saw that I couldn't stop shaking, she took off her shoes and got into the shower with me, clothes and all. I was dumbstruck.

"When she was helping me to dry off, I asked her why she did that, get into the shower to help me. 'Because I love you, darling, that's why.' It wasn't just the words. It was what she did that meant so much more."

It was late Saturday afternoon, January 9, 1971, when a fire broke out at Lee Street. It apparently started in the dining room and rapidly spread through much of the downstairs and into the kitchen. Although there were fire extinguishers throughout the house, the efforts by some of the patients to control the fire were futile.

The fire department responded in minutes and quickly extinguished the blaze. While the most serious harm was limited to the dining room and kitchen, smoke had badly damaged the rest of the house as well.

Fortunately, there was only one patient undergoing detox at the time. He was rushed outside at the first smell of smoke. Another man upstairs climbed out a window onto the roof above the kitchen and shimmied down a drainpipe. All the women were quickly ushered out the back door while the remaining men tried to fight the blaze with the fire extinguishers. No one was injured by either the fire or the smoke.

As providence would have it, there was a big old house across the street John and Dot had purchased and refurbished as part of the hospital development project. It was to serve as a future residence for the employees who would staff the hospital, principally nurses. However, since it had not been occupied as yet, it was quickly turned into a temporary home for the Lee Street patients.

When the shock of the fire was over, there was a pause for sober reflection. The smoke had spread so rapidly that the occupants of the house had only minutes to evacuate. While no one was injured, the Lee Street experience suggested that anything short of an automatic sprinkler system would be totally inadequate for the new hospital even though the zoning codes at that time did not require it.

Both John and Dot insisted that every safety precaution be taken for the good of all the patients who would be coming to Willingway in the years ahead, despite the extra costs and the delay in finishing the building. As John once said, "We had almost finished construction when I ordered it stopped until we could arrange to have a sprinkler system installed. The Small Business Administration and our local bank were both quite annoyed with me because the delay was very costly.

"Also, our loan repayments to the SBA as well as to the bank and our private investors had been scheduled to begin with anticipated patient revenue in April of 1971. We never saw our first dollar until the end of that August. Still, all past-due interest and past-due notes were paid by August of 1974. Willingway remained current from that point on."

It was serendipity once again that construction of the hospital was completed about the same time that all the repairs and remodeling work on Lee Street were finished. The remaining patients were transferred to Willingway, and John and Dot had a home all to themselves once again.

Willingway opened as a twenty-eight-bed facility with a staff of sixty full-time and part-time employees that included doctors, nurses, counselors, cooks, cleaners, and security people. As the reputation of the treatment center became more widely known and the number of patients steadily increased, the hospital had to be expanded several times.

Today Willingway is a forty-bed facility that employs more than 125 full- and part-time people. It is, in fact, one of the largest employers in Bulloch County, Georgia.

Facing a lovely private lake on thirteen beautiful, tree-covered acres, the Willingway facility includes an eight-bed detoxification unit called the "Chandelier Room" in honor of the attractive chandelier that hangs from the ceiling. It is a replica of the original chandelier that hung in the Mooney dining room at Lee Street and was put in the hospital to "keep the memory green."

There are also meeting rooms for private counseling sessions, a large conference room for talks and discussions, and an activities building with an indoor swimming pool, physical exercise equipment, and hydrotherapy facilities. Transportation is also provided to pick up new patients at airports and take them to outside recovery meetings as they near the end of their treatment.

One thing Dr. Mooney was always particularly grateful for was the opportunity he had to treat other impaired physicians sent to his hospital, and the pleasure he had in seeing so many of them stay sober. He became an integral part of the highly respected group of International Doctors in Alcoholics Anonymous. He spoke frequently at their conferences, always receiving rave reviews for his talk and his approach to handling addiction. As a result, many young physicians with an alcohol- or drug-related problem were sent to Willingway by medical groups and associations that tried to help them save their medical licenses.

The sober physician would tell his young colleagues right from the start of the treatment program he had designed that the appellation of "Doctor" would be left at the front door: "Our philosophy here at Willingway is simply this: Dr. Mooney stayed drunk, John got sober. If John stays sober, then Dr. Mooney won't get drunk. The basic person—John—must get sober. That's why we insist on first names only. No titles."

That rule also applied to every patient at the hospital, regardless of wealth, fame, or brash ego. Anonymity and confidentiality were basic tenets, and only first names were used. Both men and women were discouraged from seeking personal information from their fellow patients since most alcoholics and drug addicts treasure their privacy and fear its revelation—at least until they feel more comfortable being sober.

As for privacy, another unique aspect of the recovery facility John and Dot built was that there were no hospital wards or multi-patient rooms. Each patient had a private room. Because the Mooneys understood the sometimes unusual and complex traits of addicts—again from their own experience—the couple believed patients shouldn't be coerced into constant socializing. They felt that fellowship with others at the treatment center should happen at its own pace. So a private room allowed patients to go off on their own if they so chose after the last evening therapy session, to be alone reading or writing or simply to enjoy their own room, similar to what they were used to at home.

Other important components of the rehabilitation program at Willingway were developed through the close daily contact and experience John and Dot Mooney had with hundreds of alcoholics they had spent time with at Lee Street. For example, talking one day with a patient who had been going to AA meetings but was still getting repeatedly drunk, John asked if the man had ever written a rigorously honest account of his life. This was known in the AA program as a Fourth Step inventory. The man had not. So it was suggested that he do so before leaving treatment.

Not surprisingly, the man gained new insight into himself. That's when the Mooneys made what became known as the "Life History" a requirement for every patient. It remains to this day one of the most important parts of the therapy program at Willingway. The confidential history helps patients face those shameful and guilty feelings that had been bothering them for years, things they never dared to reveal to anyone. The patient reads it to his or her qualified counselor shortly before leaving and then burns it in front of the counselor to protect the patient's privacy.

The physician and his wife also discovered that the rate of relapse in individuals who were treated for alcoholism was very high if, after leaving, those patients used any kind of mood-altering drugs such as tranquilizers, sedatives, or stimulants—or any other medication for that matter. The Mooneys and their staff became convinced that freedom from the use of all mood-changing or habit-forming drugs would be required if the individual were to have the best chance of permanent recovery.

When once asked by a patient how he would know if he was taking a habit-forming drug, the recovered surgeon smiled.

"Well, let me put it this way," he said. "There are two kinds of pills: habit forming and non-habit forming. The habit-forming ones are the old ones and the non-habit forming ones are the new ones. When the new ones become old, they become habit forming and are replaced by new non-habit-forming ones. In other words, if you're an alcoholic, stay away from every damn pill in the drugstore."

Under the guidance of John and Dot, their counseling staff at Willingway told every new patient that they could not possibly stay sober if they took any kind of mood-altering substance—that their sobriety could best be achieved through an intensified behavioral program based upon AA's Twelve Steps to Recovery.

That's how the Mooneys and their Willingway recovery center became nationally known for using "Abstinence-Based Treatment" instead of "Medication-Based Treatment" to better assure the long-term sobriety of their patients.

John would often explain his treatment philosophy this way, and his words are as relevant today as they were then: "Practically every psychiatrist I went to for help with my alcohol and drug problem prescribed things such as Seconal, Miltown, Librium, or Valium and expected me to stay clean and sober. It didn't work. I had to learn the hard way that there are no safe, nonaddictive medications for most alcoholics and drug addicts.

"Yet there are bunches of these new so-called magic bullets being marketed all the time, and doctors are prescribing them as a big help or even a possible cure for alcoholism. They're not. In fact, most of them are very harmful over a period of time. Abstinence-based treatment is the only way for addicts to get sober. They need a clean brain to work a recovery program and also be diagnosed accurately for any other disorders they may have."

He would go on to say that when a person is taking something to help him sleep, calm him down, or pep him up, he's not really a full person.

"When I do that," the physician would explain, "I'm kind of a percentage person. Not all there. I remember my first sponsor once said to me, 'John, it don't take a whole lot of sense to get sober, but it takes all you got. So your best bet is to stop taking those things and restore your mind to full working capability.' And that's it—my full mental capacity. I could see that back then and I can see it now. So I never want to cloud my mind with those things because something bad could very well happen."

The only exceptions Dr. Mooney ever made for the use of drugs was for detoxification purposes or to treat a diagnosed mental illness. That's why, before Willingway opened in 1971, he wrote a detailed, carefully worded, six-page "Detoxification Treatment Protocol" for his staff. It contained some interesting insights and discoveries the physician had made while caring for so many alcoholics over the years. Here are some interesting excerpts from his staff memo at that time:

> Upon admission, the patient should be observed for evidences of overdosage. It is not uncommon for alcoholics to drink large quantities of alcohol or take large doses of medication just before entering a treatment center.

> While the attendants are undressing the patient and awaiting the visit of the doctor or nurse, they should watch closely for evidences of developing drowsiness. In thirty minutes or so, after vital signs have been checked and general physical condition observed, the patient should be given a test dose of a mild tranquilizer to determine his or her susceptibility to sedative medication.

> There is considerable disagreement about the choice of drugs for sedation. Any physician is probably going to make his own decision, usually based on his personal experience with various tranquilizers and sedatives. We have tried many different procedures and experimented with a variety of drugs to achieve the desired sedation. Long ago we settled on Phenobarbital. It is, in our opinion, superior to all other available preparations including the benzodiazepines for this purpose. There are many reasons.

> Phenobarbital is probably the best anticonvulsant known. The sedative effect is consistent. Paradoxical effects are nearly nonexistent. Sensitivity reactions are rare. Addiction liability is low. Discontinuance of Phenobarbital is rarely followed by depression or other rebound symptoms.

> It appears that most of the management problems associated with the treatment of acute alcoholism or acute drug addiction may be complicated by IV fluids or prescribed al-

cohol doses in reduced amounts. When these two elements are eliminated, the nursing managerial problems are usually resolved. Therefore, the first requirement of the treatment is, one, no alcohol and two, no IV fluids.

Alcohol simply prolongs the withdrawal period, increases the incidence of complications and provokes unmanageability. The use of alcohol in diminishing quantities is never desirable and can be hazardous or even disastrous. The patient is usually sufficiently saturated with alcohol when he comes in and the administration of more alcohol only aggravates the condition and delays recovery.

The average patient for detoxification may appear to be severely dehydrated. The natural reaction of a physician is to start an intravenous infusion. If the patient has been drinking very long or the amount has been fairly large, there is a good chance that the administration of 1,000 cc of liquid intravenously will be followed by severe agitation, delirium, and, perhaps convulsions.

Our experience suggests that although there is an appearance of dehydration, this is due to an altered distribution of body fluids and, actually, there is edema of the central nervous system. Giving more fluids may increase the central nervous system edema and bring on delirium and convulsions. There is no need to rush therapy for what appears to be dehydration. In time oral liquids will suffice.

Then the physician laid out some basic principles involving recovery:

a) Alcoholism is a separate and distinct disease entity.

b) Alcoholism is a total disease of the total person—body, mind and soul.

c) The goal for rehabilitation should be complete recovery.

d) Alcoholics have a peculiar susceptibility to any type of mood changing drug.

e) The personal, sociological, financial, and other problems are the results of alcoholism, not the cause.

f) The most effective agency available to help the alcoholic stop drinking is Alcoholics Anonymous.

One of the things that Dot Mooney was always proudest of was the Family Program she initiated when Willingway first opened. Much of it was based on the experience she had had attending Al-Anon Family Group meetings early on in her sobriety and also having some of her children participate in the Alateen program.

"Alcoholism and drug addiction don't only affect the alcoholic and addict," she would always say. "Those closest to them, family members in particular, get caught up in all that destructive behavior and don't know what to do about it. I know that from my own personal experience living with my husband and also watching some of my children get run over by this terrible disease.

"A wife or husband often feels guilty, ashamed, and obsessed with trying to control the alcoholic. As a result, they become almost as sick as the addict and need help to recover."

The Family Program was offered free as part of the hospital's overall treatment protocol. It was held during the last week of a patient's stay. Family members would meet for discussions with the physician and counselors, view films and videos about recovery, eat with the patients, and attend group therapy sessions. The goal was to encourage them to join a support group for themselves such as Al-Anon and continue to recover along with their addicted family member.

"We would try to make their participation in our Family Program a condition of accepting patients prior to their admission," Dot explained. "Most of the time the family member or members were so desperate they would always agree. There were times, however, when the anger and resentment that had been created by the disease would prevent that from happening. But we always kept trying."

While she enjoyed her involvement at Willingway and the good work she and her husband were doing, Dot Mooney still had that old resentment smoldering inside—the one sparked by John's lack of attention. She had thought staying busy was the solution. In fact, she convinced herself the resentment was gone. It wasn't. And every time her energetic spouse would work late at his medical practice, burn the midnight oil at the hospital, or fly off on weekends to recovery meetings, her resentment would grow just a little bit more.

Dot always cherished the few days they would spend together driving to and from out-of-town AA conventions and other gatherings—nights at motels, dinners by themselves. However, with the physician now flying most of time, even that togetherness was gone.

"One day I was talking with some of my lady friends in AA about self-honesty," she once shared. "Suddenly I realized I had stopped being honest with my husband about my true feelings. I knew he still loved me, but we were both so busy now taking care of everybody else that we were no longer communicating with each other about ourselves.

"Here we were twelve sober years together and we were becoming strangers. I got so angry at him I was ready to scream. Then I realized I was angry at him because I was so angry at myself for not telling him how I felt. But I knew I shouldn't say anything when I got that angry so I waited for the right opportunity to talk with him.

"John had been invited to speak at something called the Blackstone Retreat in Virginia and he invited me to fly there with him. I said I was too busy. That was a lie. Every time I'd fly with him, I couldn't hear anything over the loud noise of the engines. You couldn't talk. I thought if I went, he'd be sitting there flying that damned airplane and me sitting there madder than hell. I just didn't want to go with him that way.

"Later that night John came into the bedroom and found me crying like a baby. He sat down next to me, put his arm around me, and asked what was wrong. That was the night I surrendered to my pride and became totally honest with him. I said, 'John, I can't go on like this. I don't have you anymore. Everybody else does. I need you to spend more time with me. Please, John. I love you.'

"He pulled me close and said, 'You know how much I love you too. Why didn't you just tell me how you felt? I need you too.'

"I climbed onto his lap and we just sat there hugging and rocking for a long time."

The next day John and Dot drove to the Blackstone Retreat. They stayed at fine motels both going and coming and enjoyed having dinner together just by themselves.

When they returned home, the physician sat down with his nurse, Dallas Cason, and told her to start notifying all his patients that he would be closing his medical practice and, if they would like him to, he would suggest other doctors they could see for their medical needs. He would only be working at Willingway from then on.

John went home to his wife that afternoon and sat with her to plan their first vacation together in many years.

CHAPTER FIFTEEN

A Family Legacy

THE FIRST PATIENT ADMITTED TO WILLINGWAY HOSPITAL WHEN its doors finally opened on August 12, 1971, was not an alcoholic or a drug addict. However, the reason for his admittance was directly related to the disease of alcoholism.

Willingway's first patient was, strangely enough, John and Dot's oldest son, Al, who had almost been killed by a drunken driver on his way back to medical school one night. As Al explained, "I was engaged at that time to my wife, Jane, who was studying at Agnes Scott in Atlanta. I would visit her on weekends, then I'd drive back to the Medical College of Georgia in Augusta where I was finishing my medical studies.

"I was cruising along I-20 in my little Volkswagen convertible when suddenly this big Chevrolet Impala comes barreling across the divide from the other side of the interstate and smashes head-on into me. I should have been killed. Instead, the drunken driver died along with his passenger in the front seat and someone in his back seat lost a leg. Anytime I begin taking life too seriously, I simply remember that I shouldn't even be here.

"I wound up with more broken bones than they could count. They had me in traction at an Atlanta hospital for more than three months before they put me in a body cast for another few months. As I began to mend, my dad asked me to come back to Statesboro so he could take care of me.

"Since I still needed to be hospitalized, he put me into Bulloch County Hospital for a few weeks until Willingway opened. Then my father smiled and said he wouldn't charge me anything if I came over to his hospital. So I did—and became the first patient to be admitted there. I not only got great medical care from a great doctor, but I also had the love and support of two wonderful parents."

As Al lay there watching very sick addicted men and women of all ages and from all walks of life being admitted for treatment, he couldn't help but think about the past and how this terrible disease had often deprived him of the time and attention of two loving parents during his growing-up years.

But that was then and this was now, and he no longer harbored the resentment he once had against his father and Alcoholics Anonymous. That had left him several years before when he and his dad found something they both loved and something that brought them very close together.

"It occurred in the spring of 1968," Al recalled, "when I was still single and still at Emory. I happened to be home the weekend my brother Jimmy got his pilot's license and soloed for the first time. It was contagious. Suddenly I was in love with flying and started coming home at every opportunity to take instructions and get my flight time. Before long I took my flight test, got my private pilot's license, and have been flying ever since.

"My dad got the flying bug at the same time, and when he would get interested in something, there was no stopping him. He not only got his pilot's license but bought his own airplane. That's when he and I began flying a lot together and spending a lot of time with each other. It was great. I remember we flew out to Denver for the International Doctors of Alcoholics Anonymous convention and to Iowa City for another big AA function.

"When my father began getting pretty sick from emphysema due to his heavy smoking, he wasn't really able to fly by himself very much. So I would fly him everywhere. Many times I'd pick him up at Willingway, drive him to the airport, fly him to his AA talk, stay while he gave his talk, and often we'd fly back together the same night. I must have listened to him give his AA talk more than a hundred times.

"And that became very important to me even though I was the only one in the family who didn't become an alcoholic or drug addict. It finally helped me get over my resentment against him and AA because I realized as I listened to him speak, telling his story over and over again, how important recovery and the AA program were to him and also the opportunities and the decent life it had given me."

It wasn't long before all the beds at Willingway were filled with alcoholics badly in need of treatment—a councilwoman from Savannah; a retail liquor dealer from Little Rock, Arkansas; a lady sales clerk from Alma, Georgia; a surgeon from Charlotte, North Carolina; a railway engineer from Atlanta; and a business executive from Jacksonville, Florida. There was also a criminal attorney, a construction engineer, the manager of a cigar company, a doctor of internal medicine, a shoe salesman, and a housewife. The youngest patient was fourteen and the oldest was eighty-seven.

"The diversity among the patients only emphasized the fact that the disease of alcoholism can affect anyone," Dot would always comment. "Whether they're young or old, rich or poor, black or white, male or female.

"I'll never forget this one young woman who arrived at Willingway in a chauffeur-driven limousine. She came from a very wealthy family and had never worked a day in her life. We learned she had grown up with butlers and maids, went to private schools and had tutors, yet by the time she was a teenager, she was a full-blown alcoholic and drug addict.

"She'd been an alcoholic for more than fifteen years before she was sent to us by a psychiatrist in Florida. The lady was married but separated from her husband, who had gone off to Europe. She had been in and out of many treatment places, so we said we wouldn't accept her unless she agreed to stay until we thought she was well enough to leave. Being very sick physically and drained emotionally, she agreed. I felt she was finally ready to do something about her problem.

"Believe it or not, the young woman actually stayed with us almost two years. She not only got sober but finally began to think about her life in a mature way. She and I would talk about what she'd like to do once she left Willingway. As a young girl, she used to dream about becoming a nurse. Now, watching the wonderful nurses on our staff, she made up her mind to go into nursing.

"Being financially well off, the young woman got an apartment in Savannah, became actively involved in Alcoholics Anonymous, went into nurse's training, and became an LPN. She returned to her home in Florida and today is helping other people get well."

Dot said she always felt a great deal of gratitude for being allowed to play a role in the recovery of such people. She was also very grateful for being able to do it alongside her husband each day at their new hospital.

"While I kind of hated to pack away my scalpel and forceps and close my medical office about a year after we started Willingway," John once shared, "I quickly came to realize it was all for the best—not just for Dot and me and our relationship, but for our patients as well. It seemed only fitting that I spend my remaining years in medicine treating alcoholics and drug addicts since the disease of addiction came pretty close to being the death of me."

Most people who came to the treatment center at the beginning were alcoholics, although the hospital was fully equipped and staffed to care for the most seriously ill drug addicts. John was always quite forceful and direct when discussing both the similarities and the differences between alcoholism and drug addiction.

"Since alcohol is a drug," he would say, "just as heroin and morphine are, people who abuse alcohol can easily become drug abusers, and the reverse is also true. However, there is an important distinction.

"Alcohol is relatively inexpensive and can be purchased almost anywhere since it is a legal drug. Heroin and similar drugs are not. Also, a person on heroin has to get into crime, unless he owns an oil well. And a girl hooked on drugs almost has to become a prostitute. What else can she do if she's not independently wealthy? She can't work and she will do anything to support her habit.

"Law enforcement can force people to accept treatment as an alternative to going to jail, which can be good. I've always believed that some kind of outside pressure on addicted people can help get them to face their problem which is exactly what happened to me."

Then he would conclude by explaining that Willingway was set up to treat all drug dependency problems the same way.

"This is a general medical problem. We know it's a disease and that it can be treated. We discourage looking for why a person becomes an alcoholic or drug addict. We advocate a program of honesty and responsibility, a willingness to look at ourselves honestly, which is the only pathway to recovery."

One of the physician's deepest concerns had always been that once a sober patient left treatment, he or she could relapse if given almost any kind of narcotic or pharmaceutical drug for a prolonged period of time.

For example, John feared that someone undergoing surgery might be prescribed a painkiller or tranquilizer upon discharge by a doctor who didn't fully understand the complexities of addiction. So all sober patients leaving Willingway were given a special letter for their surgeons should they require an operation of any type. Here are some of the important excerpts from that letter:

Dear Doctor:

When I was a patient in rehab, they told me there is often a misconception about the meaning of "dangerous medication." They said that doctors think of "hard drugs" like morphine, Dilaudid, Pantopon, and Demerol as being dangerous and "mild" drugs like tranquilizers as being safe. In a way, the staff said, this is backwards. The hard narcotics given for a short time to relieve pain are pretty safe, except in rare cases, while the milder drugs given by prescription over a longer period, are what's dangerous.

According to them, you can give just about any alcoholic or addict a hard drug in the same doses you give your non-alcoholic and non-addictive patients after surgery without fear of serious consequences if you stop it in three or four days.

They said the trouble comes from changes in attitude caused by the effect of the chemical on the brain. My sobriety depends upon a clear head. The few days I get the narcotic when I am still recovering from the anesthetic probably won't bother me very much but the longer usage of the prescription drug can cause a drastic change in my attitude toward everything. I will explain what I mean.

Several days after surgery when I am feeling better, I might tell you that I don't need any more strong shots and I might try to persuade you to let me go home with a prescription for a mild pain reliever that I can take if I really need it. My argument could be convincing as I am a pretty good con artist.

I might talk about how you might need the hospital bed. You might decide that maybe that's a fine idea and give me a prescription for some capsules with a little codeine or maybe some tranquilizers for nervousness and perhaps something to sleep.

Wait! Think it through!

When I get a prescription, I become my own doctor. If the directions say to take one pill four times a day, I might decide that it would be the same if I just waited until night and then took four at one time. In a few days I will probably want a refill. If you are out of town, I will call another doctor. I might claim the medicine you gave me had been lost through "calamities." I can say that the dog got it or the car ran over it or it was flushed accidentally down the toilet.

Remember, I am operating under compulsion and I just might get more of that drug somewhere regardless of what it takes. You see, by then, my sanity is gone and I am in a chemical fantasy land. I may not yet be drunk, but it's probably only a matter of time.

Please prevent this if you can. Please don't send me home with any prescriptions.

Sincerely,

Your surgical patient for tomorrow.

Patients would often call Willingway after their surgery and thank their counselor or one of the nurses for the letter, which they said opened an understanding dialogue with their doctor. On occasion, a physician or surgeon would call to discuss the letter and its implications.

For many years, John and Dot Mooney believed that what they did at their Lee Street home and what they were doing now at Willingway was simply practicing the Twelfth Step of the Alcoholics

Anonymous program in their lives: "Having had a spiritual awakening as the result of these steps, we tried to carry this message to
alcoholics and to practice these principles in all our affairs."

In other words, this is the way AA suggests that one alcoholic
try to help another alcoholic find sobriety. And this is what the
physician and his wife believed they were doing—simply working
the Twelfth Step in their lives.

It wasn't until the fall of 1973, when John was having lunch
one day with his good friend and accountant Earl Dabbs, that he
began to see his role in helping others recover from alcoholism in
a much different way.

The hospital was beginning its third year of operations. While
John had often expressed his gratitude to the man who helped
make it all possible, they were both always so busy that he had
never taken the time out to sit down with Earl, look him in the
eye, and thank him sincerely for Willingway's great success at saving so many lives and restoring so many families. So he invited
him to lunch.

"John got so emotional I was afraid he was going to cry in his
soup," the accountant joshed as he recalled that special afternoon.
"He told me how much he appreciated everything I did for him. I
tried to explain that my business was finance and his business was
medicine and it simply turned out to be an excellent partnership.
He just wanted me to know that as far as he was concerned, it was
much more than that. And I understood."

But then when his doctor friend remarked that the hospital
was enabling him to expand his Twelve-Step work, the accountant, who knew little about the workings of AA, stopped him and
said, "No, John. You're not doing Twelve-Step work. You're doing
far more than that. If all your patients needed was Twelve-Step
work, they can get sober just by going to AA meetings like you
did and they wouldn't have to go to Willingway."

That's when a lightbulb clicked on in the physician's head. He
went back to his office that afternoon, took the AA Big Book off

the shelf, and turned to the opening paragraph of Chapter Five. It read:

> Rarely have we seen a person fail who has thoroughly followed our path. Those who do not recover are people who cannot or will not completely give themselves to this simple program, usually men and women who are constitutionally incapable of being honest with themselves. There are such unfortunates. They are not at fault; they seem to have been born that way.
>
> They are naturally incapable of grasping and developing a manner of living that demands rigorous honesty. Their chances are less than average. There are those, too, who suffer from grave emotional and mental disorders, but many of them do recover if they have the capacity to be honest.

As he reread those words several times over, the physician began to see more clearly what they actually meant. The first sentence of the paragraph explained just how AA worked—by thoroughly following the path of those who found sobriety. The rest of the paragraph explained how AA didn't work and for whom it didn't work—those who were incapable of being honest with themselves.

"As a physician," John often said, "I had always struggled with why some alcoholics needed someone like me when all the answers to sobriety can be found right there in Alcoholics Anonymous just as they were for me. But now I understood the difference.

"I always knew there had to be more to treatment than just getting very sick people dried out and physically well. Once you get the alcohol and drugs out of their system through detox, that's when the real work begins. By helping people find a way to get honest with themselves and others, we are getting them ready to be 12-stepped into the AA program where they can engage with others like themselves in lifelong recovery."

John Mooney now had another reason to be grateful to Earl

Dabbs—for helping him to a better understanding of what was really behind the work he and his wife were doing at Willingway and how it truly related to the fellowship of Alcoholics Anonymous. But little did he know that his accountant would soon have another reason for being grateful to the physician.

"I remember once saying to John," Earl explained, "this hospital is going to be a real nice place when we finish it, but I hope I never have to use it. I wound up eating those words, although I was happy to do so."

One of Earl's close family members became seriously addicted to alcohol and drugs. Fortunately, when the family member was ready to do something about the problem, Earl and John had built Willingway. The relative was treated there by John and Dot and went on to live a sober and successful life.

"Like my wonderful friend Dr. Mooney always used to say," Earl commented, "God works in strange ways."

Ironically, there was another good friend of John's who also became seriously alcoholic and needed the help and care Willingway offered. He was Jay Cason, the husband of Dallas Cason, the nurse who supported the once-addicted physician through her loyalty and dedication over the years.

"It's funny sometimes how things work out," Dallas remarked. "When Dr. Mooney was so sick from all his drinking and drugging, my husband would drive me to his house and help me take care of him. Then Jay got worse and worse himself from his alcoholism. He would even drive drunk, which was when I finally put my foot down. So once he was ready to do something about his problem, Dr. Mooney was there to help him."

The experienced nurse also continued to be there for her friend and boss, working both at his medical office and helping at Lee Street. And when Willingway opened and John decided to commit himself full time to the hospital, Dallas was right there beside him.

In setting up the facility and hiring employees, there were

many times when Dallas would be the only nurse and would have to spend the night at the hospital. Meanwhile, she had three daughters of her own to care for, but fortunately she still had that kind and loving mother-in-law to help her.

As more nurses were hired and the hospital's reputation grew, Dot asked her dear friend Dallas to become the director of nursing, which she did. She set up the pharmacy and established the policies and procedures for the nursing department.

Although she was busy with all this work, the always generous nurse still found time to visit with and talk to patients.

"One of the sad changes I've seen in nursing over the years," she commented, "is that nurses get so busy dealing with rules and regulations and supporting the doctors that they don't have enough time for direct patient care. My greatest reward has always been my interaction with patients, seeing their lives change from something that's 'going down the tubes' to a life that's hopeful and meaningful."

Dallas said she knew from the beginning that Willingway would help many people recover from the disease of alcoholism, especially when she saw her own husband get well and stay sober for the rest of his life. And there was still another incident she liked to recall that underscored the hospital's importance even more.

"I was speaking with this new patient one morning," she said, "and noticed he had a slightly different accent. He said he was from Toronto, Canada, and I was taken aback a bit. Naturally I asked how he managed to find his way to Statesboro, Georgia.

"He said he was having coffee one morning in this small Toronto restaurant and his hands were trembling so much he was spilling his coffee. A man at the next table told him he once had the same problem when he lived in the States. He told the fellow if he really wanted to do something about his problem, he should go to a place called Willingway in Statesboro, Georgia—that they could get anybody sober. So he came.

"That's what Willingway is all about—helping people at the

end of their road. We offer them love and hope. We put an arm around them and say we understand what you're going through and we're going to help you."

The caring nurse said she would always have fond memories of Dr. Mooney, a man she respected as a doctor despite his addictions and a man she came to admire greatly for his unselfish dedication to helping others.

She summed it up this way: "When I first met Dr. John Mooney, he was a good doctor doing his best to take care of other people. If he needed something to get him by, he took it. That's the way he cured his own ills, by taking a drink. And then he got sicker and sicker and finally had to do something about it. He did, and he changed to a completely different and much more caring person.

"He said to me one day that he had spent the first half of his life selfishly taking care of himself and hoped to spend the last half of his life helping to take care of other sick alcoholics. I think there are thousands of them grateful to him for that."

When John gave up his medical practice and began keeping more regular hours at Willingway, both he and Dot expected that time to be the most contented and perhaps the happiest period of their lives. It might well have been except for the undeniable evidence that three of their four children were having all sorts of problems—and the problems were getting increasingly worse. Jimmy, Bobby, and Carol Lind were all failing either at school, at work, or in their relationships.

Reluctantly, their parents were forced to accept that the addictions that had nearly destroyed their own lives were now threatening to destroy those of their children. Instead of being a time of joy, it turned out to be one of the most painful periods they had to face.

Jimmy was the first of their offspring to start drinking and the last to get sober. In each case, their parents were slow to catch on since the siblings were very clever at hiding their habits. But the one thing both John and Dot sadly knew from their own experience was that their children would have to hit some kind of "bottom" to bring about a desire for recovery. It was heartbreaking for them to accept that they were powerless to help their own children.

Bobby Mooney said he began abusing alcohol and drugs at age twelve and continued all through school. He married early, left home to go to college in Rochester, New York, separated from his wife, and came back to Statesboro, where, struggling to hide his drinking and drugging, he actually went to work at Willingway, creating video and photographic presentations for patient education.

Talking with addicts in detox, he soon realized that many of them sounded just like him. Bobby could identify with what they said and how they thought. Then he witnessed in a matter of weeks these same people looking and sounding much better while he was just the same or worse. So, at the age of twenty-four, he began thinking seriously about suicide.

"There was hardly a day," Bobby said, "that I did not think of ending my life. I hated myself and everyone around me. My alcohol and drug use had eaten a dark hole into my soul, and it finally got to the point that one day I was driving across a bridge and thought to myself, 'If I turn this wheel just a little I won't have to hurt anymore.' I was so frightened by the thought that I became willing to do something I had never been willing to do before—reach out for help. I had grown up surrounded by recovery and now I wanted it for myself. My recovery today depends upon my willingness to continue to ask for help, and I pray that I never forget what my life was like before sobriety."

The Mooneys' youngest son went on to attend medical school. He graduated from the Mercer University School of Medicine, received his medical license, and then completed his residency in psychiatry at East Tennessee State University. Today he is the medical director and chief psychiatrist at Willingway and is involved in recovery activities and organizations all across the country.

Jimmy Mooney also dropped out of college after suffering an early broken marriage. Like his younger brother, he too worked at Willingway for a short time, running outside every chance he got to hide behind some tall trees and smoke pot. He also did some farming for a while but found the hard work interfered too much with his drinking and drugging.

He finally hit bottom during a motorcycle trip with some friends to Daytona Beach. Along the way, the group stopped several times to drink booze and use drugs. Jimmy's memory of the trip is of driving his bike at ninety miles an hour in traffic while he was completely stoned. The trip turned out to be his "miracle," his return to sanity. He came home in one piece, but he was sick of the way he was living and ready to give up his addictions.

He returned to college, graduated from Georgia Southern University with a business degree, and today oversees all the operations and activities at Willingway.

Carol Lind, the youngest in the family, was given her first drink at the age of twelve by her brother Jimmy, whom she idolized. Her first experience with drugs happened at school when a classmate offered her some pills. She says she swallowed them without even knowing what they were.

She married at sixteen but soon divorced and began mainlining drugs. After a stay at a treatment center in New Jersey, she returned to Statesboro and almost immediately began drinking and drugging again. Her mother finally put her foot down, telling her daughter she could come home for a meal but couldn't stay unless she decided to do something serious about her problem.

Totally powerless over her addictions at that point, Carol Lind moved into a tent by the railroad tracks that she shared with her boyfriend. The two collected soda cans to get money to feed their habits. Often the young woman would wind up in the emergency room at Bulloch County Hospital after overdosing on alcohol and drugs.

There seemed to be no hope. But then Carol Lind finally hit bottom too. Something happened that turned her around. She said she simply woke up one morning after another heavy night of swilling down booze and mainlining drugs and had this deep, burning desire to be sober. She said her last drunk had been no better or no worse than any other, yet something powerful had happened to her as a result. She believes it was a gift from God, and she has been clean and sober ever since.

The Mooneys' daughter also went back to school, graduating from Georgia Southern University in 1991 with a BS in psychology. She then went to Mercer Law School and graduated from there in 1995 with her law degree. Carol Lind has worked for the State Bar of Georgia helping impaired lawyers, has set up and supervised drug courts, and today runs recovery homes for alcoholic and drug-addicted women, among her many other activities.

Her oldest brother, Al, is the only Mooney sibling who never became addicted. He also never intended to work in the field of addiction treatment, the way everyone else in the family did. His ambition was to be a surgeon like his dad.

However, while assisting in the operating room during his medical training, Al saw that too often the root cause of a gunshot or knife wound or other forms of family violence that brought patients to the hospital was usually related to substance abuse. This was also true of many car accidents, such as the one that almost killed him. So, after getting his medical license, he returned to Statesboro and, when his father became ill, he took over as the medical director of Willingway for a number of years.

Concerning her children's problems with addiction, Dot explained: "It was difficult for John and me to deal with our children's alcoholism. It was especially difficult for me because of all my false pride. I was telling somebody the other day that when they were drinking and wearing hippie clothes and long hair and ponytails, it was embarrassing.

"I remember when someone would ask how they were all doing, I'd say my son Al is doing wonderful. He's flying airplanes, he's becoming a surgeon. He's doing this and doing that. Al is just great. Then I'd hurry off before they could ask me how my other kids were doing.

"I had a hard time with that because, despite my own earlier drinking and drugging, I put a lot of work into trying to bring these children up right and make them wear decent clothes and look decent. My pride was hurt and I couldn't tell anybody. I'd just act like everything was all right and avoid talking about them any way I could.

"I've had to work through all of this. I've had to recognize my own character defects in all of this. I learned to 'Let go and let God.' I had to go to Al-Anon to work on it. And thank God for Al-Anon. I don't think I would be here if it weren't for Al-Anon. In fact I'm sure of it.

"The Al-Anon program was of particular help in my relationship with my daughter. I remember leaving a meeting one night and realizing in my heart and accepting in my soul that I had to be willing to let Carol Lind go. I had to be willing to let her die if that was necessary. And I knew it was a big risk. But I also knew I was powerless to do anything about it. So I did what Al-Anon suggested I do. I knelt down and said, 'God, she's all yours. I am totally powerless. Please help my Carol Lind. I can't say I felt any better right away but I knew then that God would take care of her. And He did.'"

When once asked why it took them some time to become aware of their children's addictions, Dot's husband commented: "Sometimes we only see what we want to see."

One of the important things that John always saw, however, was how the stigma of addiction killed people. The fear of someone "finding out" discouraged many people from seeking help and also encouraged families to "cover up" the shame by denying they had an alcoholic or drug addict in their homes. The physician was always trying to find ways to reduce that fear and shame.

That's why he accepted an invitation from the National Council on Alcoholism to participate in an event called "Operation Understanding" held in Washington, D.C., on May 8, 1976. It was aimed at eradicating the stigma associated with alcoholism. John, together with fifty-two other well-known men and women from all walks of life, including astronaut Buzz Aldrin, actor Dick Van Dyke, TV host Gary Moore, politicians, sports figures, and business executives, stood up at a major press conference and told the world they were recovered alcoholics.

The event had no affiliation with Alcoholics Anonymous. No one who was in AA revealed their membership and therefore did not break the Fellowship's tradition of anonymity. But their declaration was heard around the world and did much to reduce the stigma of addiction.

It was around 1980 when John's many years of heavy cigarette smoking finally began to take their toll. While he had stopped smoking several years before, he had already developed emphysema, which led to a breathing condition called COPD—chronic obstructive pulmonary disease. He was put on various medications to treat his lungs and to help his breathing.

He tried at first to make light of it. In fact, when he had severe coughing spells during his regular group counseling sessions with patients, he would tell them jokingly, "I have what's called COPD, which means a charming, overwhelming, personality development."

But it got worse. His son Bobby recalled one particularly serious incident that was soon to become commonplace.

"My dad and I were in Atlanta together walking down a street. He had just quit smoking but was still having a hard time with it. He still had the urge to smoke.

"I remember kidding him about the best way to quit smoking cigarettes. I said you switch to smoking pot and then you can get treated for that. He started to laugh, and then he started to cough. We'd walk twenty feet and he'd lean up against a building and cough again. He just kept coughing and coughing and coughing. I thought he was going to die. It was one of the most horrible experiences I've ever had with my dad."

John and Dot had now built a new house closer to the hospital with all the rooms on one floor. This made it easier for the physician to get around. They called the place "Cornerstone." Since he was starting to have difficulty walking much of a distance, he began traveling around in a golf cart. He also was losing weight and required oxygen so frequently that he had a pulmonary specialist implant a revolutionary device called a transtracheal catheter that provided him with supplemental oxygen.

As his illness progressed, John spent less time treating and counseling patients and more time with his family and friends.

"In a sense," Bobby remarked, "it turned out to be a really special time, a period long enough for my dad and me to do some things together and get closer than we had ever been. Just to get to hang around with him, to let him know how grateful I was for the opportunity he gave me to understand and appreciate the importance of being sober. That was the true legacy he left me."

Carol Lind was grateful that she had found sobriety a year and a half before her father became seriously ill. She had remarried and had an infant son she named Ross.

"Every time my mom went off somewhere to speak," the Mooneys' daughter explained, "I would stay with my dad and take care of him. We had a lot of warm, warm times together and spoke about things that have helped me throughout my life.

"My daddy just loved little Ross, so I would bring my baby to Cornerstone every chance I had. I'll never forget one afternoon when my daddy had Ross cradled in his arms. He looked over at me with tears in his eyes and said, 'You know, honey, Ross is the only person in the world I can relate to right now. He's totally dependent on somebody else for almost everything he needs just like I am.'

"I went over, put my arms around him, and hugged him for a long, long time."

After John had the transtracheal catheter implanted, he started to feel somewhat better. He had been turning down requests to speak at large functions all across the country, fearing his weakened condition would prove to be a hardship or at least an inconvenience for his hosts. However, when he was invited to speak at an AA convention at nearby St. Simons Island on March 2, 1983, he decided to accept since it was so close to home. It turned out to be his last AA talk.

"For the past nine or ten months, maybe even longer, I've been sitting in my living room all alone with only old John Mooney for company and it got pretty boring," he told his AA friends from the podium that night with a big smile on his face. "I've had a lot of time to just think about me and my responsibilities and what I've been doing about them, and I came up short.

"I've spent so much time in my life trying to manage and direct other people that I neglected to take adequate care of myself in almost every department. I have this oxygen tube in me because of my physical neglect, and I'm far from the sharpest tack in the box because my mental processes have slowed down from sitting on my brains.

"Still, I'm grateful tonight because all of you have always reminded me that there's one thing I can never afford to neglect and that's my relationship with my Higher Power. God still gives me the knowledge and the strength to make changes in my life. He has taken me out of the grips of a debilitating, fatal illness for now and put me back up here on this stand where I can share my life with you.

"I feel like I'm an AA member again tonight. I feel like I'm one of you. And it's the first time I've really felt that way in some time. And I want to thank you for inviting me here, for listening, and for God giving me the privilege of being here. I love you, and God bless you all."

The last few years of John's life were difficult for all concerned, especially for Dot. Her husband's breathing was not his only problem. He was dying of congestive heart failure. She once said that

period was harder than she ever thought she could have survived. But again, the program and the fellowship of Alcoholics
Anonymous didn't let her down. It gave her the friendship, courage, strength, and support she needed—together with a pattern
for living and a pattern for dying.

Always nearby were close friends like Lou Vasser, who was a
women's counselor at Willingway; Corliss Gibbons, who had been a
patient at Lee Street; and Joe and Shirley Wallace, whom she knew
from the first day she sobered up. So were Dallas Cason, Nancy
Waters, and all of Dot and John's now sober and caring children.

By the end of October 1983, Dr. John Mooney was mostly bedridden. It was close to the end. Dot once shared those final days
and that final morning hour of November 10, 1983.

"I was so very tired," she said. "I had brought nurses in from
time to time to stay with him so I could get some sleep. He didn't
sleep much because of the pain in his back. But this day was different. I knew the time was close, but I was so tired. That night I
said, 'Honey, I feel like I need to get a nurse to stay with you tonight so I can get some rest.' And he said, 'No, I want you to get
in this bed and sleep with me just like you've always done.'

"I knew he really wanted me near him. Always before, we'd go
to sleep and at about four in the morning, he would get restless
and his body would jerk. I'd wake him up and tell him to turn
over, and he'd go back to sleep.

"And so that night he started to toss around as usual. I remember looking at the clock. It was four a.m. I reached over and
touched him and said, 'Honey, why don't you turn over so you
can rest?' And he said, 'That's funny. They just called me. They
told me that I'd finished what I had to do and that I'd done a
good job. Now you wake me up and tell me to turn over and rest,
so I think that's what I'm going to do.' And he turned over and
went to sleep.

"At six, I woke up and missed his breathing. I knew right away
what had happened. He hadn't moved. His hand was under his

cheek just like he was asleep. When the doctor came, he told me he had been dead about two hours. So he died at four, right after he turned over.

"What I had dreaded most was the prospect of him having to watch us watch him die. I didn't think he could do that, and he didn't have to. It was . . . it was just a spiritual thing. His funeral was spiritual too. There were people coming and going, laughing and crying. We had a meeting right there at the house that night. We laughed and cried again and it was all very spiritual.

"John loved me. He had always loved me. But as long as I lived in the shadow of fear and suspicion, I couldn't believe it. But I waited for my miracle, and it didn't let me down. He loved me right to the very end.

"Alcoholics Anonymous is the greatest thing that's ever happened to us. We are privileged to have this program to live by— and to die by."

Dot's son Jimmy well remembers the day his father passed away.

"He'd be worse one day and then feel a little better the next," he said, recalling those last days. "I was still at the university, so it was difficult to keep tabs on things. One day I stopped by Willingway and Dr. Bill Gray, who was taking care of my father, happened to be there.

"I remember he pulled me aside and said, 'You need to see your dad. He doesn't have much time left.' So I went over to Cornerstone and sat with him for a while. He was breathing heavily, so we couldn't talk very much. He died early the next morning.

"I'm really glad I saw him before he passed away because when I went back to the house the next day and saw so many people there, I just couldn't hang around. I ended up going to class. I'm not sure why. Maybe I just wanted to get my mind off what was going on at the time. Naturally I was there for my mother and the family at the funeral.

"I look back now and regret I didn't spend more time to really get to know my father. I mean, I knew him as my dad, but when he got sick, we wasted too much time talking about superficial things like baseball and stuff. I should have talked to him more about his recovery, what it meant to him, how it changed his life like it was beginning to change mine. Still, I feel his spirit at Willingway every day I'm there."

Dr. John Mooney had just turned seventy-three. It was indeed quite appropriate that this hero of World War II should pass away on Veterans Day, November 10, 1983. The news of his death was prominently displayed on the front page of the *Statesboro Herald* right beneath a large photo of the American flag and a brief editorial honoring all those who had served in the armed forces.

The story of his passing highlighted the physician's career in the Eighty-Second Airborne Division and the medals he had won along with his career in medicine and all the honors heaped on him for his great achievements, especially in the field of addiction.

The newspaper noted that he was not only the first recipient of the Georgia Addiction Counselors Association's Distinguished Service Award, but also that the award was now known as the John Mooney Distinguished Service Award.

It seemed as if the whole city of Statesboro turned out for his funeral. John's good friend Dr. Jack Averitt was not only deeply moved by his passing but also greatly pleased that so many others also recognized the important role this physician had played in their lives. He was truly, as the professor had told himself years before, "a man worth saving."

"How do you describe a man who achieved such greatness after suffering such failure," the professor wrote in his journal. "The effectiveness of his leadership in the rehabilitation of alcoholics and drug addicts became known throughout the country and around the world.

"Dr. Mooney was called upon to speak nationally and internationally about something that was becoming one of the major problems facing the medical profession—the plague of alcoholism and drug addiction. He helped educate the world of medicine and the general public that addiction is not a social immorality but an illness—a serious medical problem that could be treated successfully so that people could resume normal lives.

"His is a story of success, not of mere achievement. It is one of outstanding success. I can say that because I witnessed it personally almost from the very beginning."

Following her husband's passing, Dot was showered with sympathy cards and letters for quite some time, along with phone calls and people dropping by. And she was rarely without the company of AA friends. However, as time passed, the realization that the man she loved so deeply and so passionately would no longer be there for her, would no longer share her bed at night or make her coffee in the morning, began to take its toll.

"I had a very hard time adjusting to living alone after thirty-six years of marriage," she once told a very close friend. "I felt so lonely at times I was scared I'd go crazy not having John to put his arms around me. I knew it would take time to get over these feelings, so I gave myself a year. I said I wouldn't do anything or make any big decisions until I could get back in touch with my real feelings.

"I went through a lot of grief and a whole lot of anger because I'd spend time thinking about all the things John and I planned to do and never did. But then I gradually began to think about all the wonderful things we did get to do together. We had a good life. We had a good relationship. We had as good a marriage as anybody could have when it came out of something that looked absolutely, totally hopeless at the beginning."

Dot's self-imposed year of nondecision was shortened by her growing desire to return to Willingway. She began to realize that was where John would want her to be. So she soon found herself back at the treatment facility as the head women's counselor. And she found it to be the answer to her grief and the path to finding her own emotional stability.

"There's nothing that can solve your own problems better than working with another alcoholic," she believed. "Besides, being back at Willingway kept me closer to John."

After her husband's passing, she and her daughter drew even closer together. Carol Lind clearly remembered what it was like when her mother took over the reins at the treatment facility.

"While she continued to do a lot of counseling for the women there," her daughter said, "my mother really began to run the place like my father did. Yes, Mama took charge.

"I remember sitting in on a board meeting one day when one of the new doctors there suggested something my mother felt was against the way she and my dad always did things. She stood up and said, 'If we can't do this according to our principles, then by God, we won't do it at all. I'm just not willing to do it. We can shut down the place and do something else.'

"She was that set on her philosophy of what was right and what was wrong. That's how she lived her life. She didn't compromise on important things. That's something she taught me—to have a value system and live by it."

There were some people, even among Dot's friends, who thought it had always been her and John's dream to have a treatment center and care for very sick alcoholics. She would explain at every opportunity that it was not the case—that she had many dreams and wishes for her life but treating drunks was not one of them.

"John and I did not have any idea when we got sober that we would end up treating alcoholics," she often shared at AA meetings. "In fact, that was something we never, ever thought about. It just happened.

"I've said many times that when you turn your will and your life over to the care of God, hang on because you never know what's going to happen. I know now that's what He wanted us to do.

"Treating alcoholics and drug addicts is not an easy job. There are times when you can get really uptight about it. So you just make more AA meetings. But it's something I've come to love, especially because it's something John and I did together."

Her oldest son, Al, said he enjoyed serving as medical director of Willingway during the time his mother was essentially running the day-to-day activities.

"We had a special relationship, my mom and I, since I was the oldest child in the family," Al commented. "And I think she felt kind of an emotional dependence on me, especially after my father died. We worked very well together, as did my brothers and sister, who also worked at Willingway. And it remains a family affair."

Another family member who also worked at the hospital was Dot's sister-in-law, Marilyn Riggs, who by now had come to love and admire "Dr. John."

"John had changed so much since the years of his drinking and had done such wonderful things with his life," she said. "They both did. I know how hard it was on Dot when he passed away."

Marilyn was the bookkeeper at Willingway for many years and became one of Dot's most trusted friends.

"When she got sick," Marilyn explained, "she asked me to help her with a lot of her personal stuff, like writing out her checks, handling her banking and personal finances, stuff like that. None of us knew how sick she was at first because her doctor kept saying she had something called fibromyalgia. It turned out to be much worse than that.

"I'm still so proud of them—proud of what they did and how they dedicated their lives to helping other people. They found out what life should be all about for all of us."

Dot Mooney ran Willingway with love and care for almost ten years after her husband passed away. She continued to expand the treatment center's reputation for excellence through her many talks about recovery all across the country. And, like her husband, she received many honors and accolades for her work from people like Betty Ford, actress Mercedes McCambridge, Marty Mann, founder of the National Council on Alcoholism, and even from the cofounder of Al-Anon herself, Lois Wilson, a lady she came to know and love.

By the beginning of 2003, Marilyn Riggs wasn't the only one concerned about Dot's growing physical problems. So were all her children. Even she herself sensed it was more than fibromyalgia. For a while she blamed all the pain she was experiencing throughout her body on her crippling arthritis. But her bones were starting to ache severely and she couldn't understand why it was happening.

"I was encouraging her to get more tests," Al Mooney said, "but my mother was a very strong-willed person who controlled her own medical life. But it seemed to me like her primary physician labeled her with the term fibromyalgia and all the other doctors she went to for second opinions kind of checked their brains at the door and didn't think she could have anything else."

But she did.

As her friends and family would tell you, Dot Mooney was never a wimp. She could withstand a great deal of pain. But by the fall of 2003, the pain was getting so intense that she told her primary doctor she was going to the Mayo Clinic in Jacksonville, Florida, for some more tests. He decided to do a PET scan to take with her. The physician was both shocked and embarrassed when the scan clearly showed his patient had cancer in her bones that was metastasizing to other parts of her body.

At the Mayo Clinic they did a series of biopsies that evidenced she had gastric cancer that had spread to her lymph glands and was also around her aorta. They started chemotherapy treatments, which made her so sick she asked to have them stopped. That's when the doctors at the clinic said she had about six months to live.

"The news came as a real blow," her youngest son, Bobby, remarked, "but like my father, it gave all her children the time to spend with her before she left us. I would go over to the house and talk with her and always came away with some good advice."

Bobby's brother Jimmy totally agreed. "She could tell you something you didn't want to hear, and you knew she was saying it with love because she cared so deeply. She just had this unique ability to cut to the core of what the true problem was and talk with you about it with love and no anger. That's why I always felt comfortable talking to her about my problems, even in those final days."

A few years after John had passed away, Dot decided to purchase a small country house overlooking the Ogeechee River. It was in a place she had always loved ever since she was a young "country girl." She would often spend time there with two of her dearest friends, Joe and Shirley Wallace from Tennessee. They had grown very close since the time Shirley had been a patient at Willingway in 1970 and Dot had been her counselor. Joe had also developed a warm relationship with John since they were both army war veterans.

It seemed like Joe and Shirley were always at Dot's side as she grew sicker and sicker during the fall of 2003. They almost became like second parents to the Mooney children, who deeply appreciated their friendship.

While Dot loved the home in Statesboro she called Cornerstone, she loved her river house even more. So when she sensed the end was drawing near, she asked Joe and Shirley and her children to take her to that lovely place on the Ogeechee River.

"We had a hospital bed put in her bedroom there," Al explained. "And we already had hospice to handle her pain and discomfort. So when she said she was ready, we all packed into cars and like a caravan, we headed for the river. Not only were Joe and Shirley with us, but also a few of my mother's other close friends.

"We carried her up to her bedroom, where she could look at the Ogeechee River she loved so much. Her whole demeanor seemed to change. If you didn't know the seriousness of her condition, you might think she would live another ten years.

"My mother died three days later, on January 7, 2004."

Carol Lind had been at a horse show in Florida with her own daughter, Sara. She didn't know how fast her mother was fading. As soon as she received a call from the family that it was only a matter of time, she rushed home and managed to make it to the river house before her mother passed away.

"When I pulled up to the river house," Carol Lind said, her eyes moist from recalling that sad moment, "I literally ran as fast as I could up the stairs and into my mother's bedroom. Al was in there with her at the time. He said, 'I'll let you spend some time with her alone,' and then he left.

"I crawled into bed with her and held her in my arms. She just looked at me and smiled. She was too weak to speak. I just told her what a wonderful job she did, what a great person she was, and that I knew she was tired and that she was going to have this great place in heaven.

"Within five minutes after I got to the river house, my mother was gone. When I came downstairs, everybody said, 'She waited on you. She waited for you to get here.' I was so grateful that she did."

Perhaps Dr. Jack Averitt, who so loved, admired, and lauded his dear friend Dr. John Mooney, best summed up the life of Dorothy Carolyn Riggs Mooney when he wrote in his journal: "Dot Mooney was an extraordinary woman who was blessed by her Creator with the gift of giving.

"I deem the most important factor in the life of this great lady was her unquenchable love for John Mooney and her determination to support him in his dedication and untiring efforts to help others.

"In her marriage commitment, she took him for better or for worse and many, many times the worst became 'worser.' But she never failed to keep that commitment.

"If there was ever a proper memorial to Dr. John Mooney, Jr. and his wife, Dot, it is already engraved in the lives of those thousands of men and women their legacy continues to save and help become useful members of society. I am so proud to have known them and to have called them my friends."

EPILOGUE

PRIOR TO HIS DEATH IN 1983, DR. JOHN MOONEY JR. REALIZED
that institutions such as Willingway could not survive on the personality of its founders alone. His hope was that the program he
and his wife built would continue to serve those in need long after
both of them were gone.

Dr. Robert Mooney explained his father's fondest desire this
way: "One of the happiest moments I saw my father experience
happened one day when he was visiting Willingway after suffering
a protracted illness. A patient approached to tell him what a wonderful place it was and asked if he knew who ran it. The patient had
no idea he was speaking with the founder. This incident confirmed
to my father that the program and institution he and my mother
created were not dependent on their personalities to endure."

In the years since it opened in 1971, Willingway has more than
survived. It has thrived despite a number of challenges that faced
the addiction field and medicine in general. Even though the
American Medical Association and the American Society of Addiction Medicine both came to recognize alcoholism as a disease,
there continues to be a pervasive stigma directed toward alcoholics and drug addicts.

Bolstered by the legacy of its founders, the Willingway staff continues to fight this stigma by providing a family-oriented, deeply caring environment. They understand that everyone with an alcohol or drug problem deserves the opportunity to find a path to hope and recovery. The determination to be of maximum service will always remain the pillar of Willingway's philosophy.

From the very beginning, the now highly acclaimed recovery center accepted patients with serious complications that even today other treatment programs are reluctant to handle. The ability to rigorously address the addiction issue that can often be masked by medical and psychiatric complications is one of the unique aspects of the Statesboro center's program.

Perhaps the most important aspect of Willingway that separates it from the thousands of other programs in the country today is its absolute commitment to an abstinence-based philosophy versus a medication-assisted program. Willingway's philosophy of complete abstinence comprises any substance that acts on the brain, including psychiatric medications and many over-the-counter substances.

Dr. John Mooney Jr. was often heard to say, "It doesn't take a lot of sense to stay sober, but it takes all you've got." His attitude toward substances continues to be the hallmark not only for those undergoing treatment but also for their families, who are included in the treatment process. Also, Willingway is one of the only such institutions that requests abstinence from all levels of staff—from the physicians, nurses, and counselors to office personnel, maintenance people, and even housekeepers.

The Mooney family, which still runs Willingway, states as one of their core principles: "The belief in abstinence is absolute and therefore everyone on our staff has to be willing to do whatever we ask our patients and their families to do."

Since the recovery center treats addiction as a family disease, family members are expected to participate in the five-day "Family Program," which is offered at no cost at the end of the inpatient treatment experience. Dot Mooney had that in mind when Willingway was initially constructed. She insisted that all the rooms in the hospital be private with a double bed and private bath so that the spouse could stay for the family program.

This total immersion for the family in the treatment experience is an advantage that most programs are unable to offer. It helps significantly, not only in the recovery from addiction, but also in the healing of relationships. As one former Willingway patient put it, "Those five days of the family program were the longest, hardest, and most wonderful days of my life. They saved our marriage."

The story of Dr. John and Dot Mooney, and the recovery program they created for Willingway, might well be summed up this way for the generations of addicts and their families yet to come. It begins with emotional pain, suffering, and remorse, and evolves for all those who desire it into a new way of life filled with joy, peace, and gratitude. After helping thousands over many years, the legacy of John and Dot Mooney and Willingway remains one of hope and inspiration.

When Two Loves Collide is set in Adobe Garamond Pro. This book was designed by Rachel Holscher. Composition by BookMobile Design and Digital Publisher Services, Minneapolis, Minnesota, and manufactured by Friesens on acid-free paper.